Geriatric Incontinence

A Behavioral and Exercise Approach to Treatment

Janet A. Hulme, M.A., P.T,

ACKNOWLEDGEMENTS

Special thanks to Barbara Penner, P.T., Gail Nevin, P.T., Linda West, R.N., Judy Mushial, R.N., Jane Stansbury, Catherine Goodman, P.T., Gayle Cochran, Pharm.D., Paul Savoca, MD, Mary Dupont, MD, Richard Billingham, MD, Carol Barnes, P.T., and the many other therapists, nurses, and physicians who have given freely of their expertise and editing prowess. I am deeply indebted to Erika and Abigail Hulme for encouragement and editing expertise. I will always appreciate all my patients that tell me what works and more importantly, what doesn't.

Geriatric Incontinence,
A Behavioral and Exercise Approach to Treatment

Copyright ©1999 by Phoenix Publishing Co.

All rights reserved, including the right to reproduce this book or portions thereof in any form or by any means, electronic or mechanical, including photocopying, recording, or by an information storage and retrieval system, without permission in writing from Phoenix Publishing Co.

ISBN Number: 1-928812-00-7

Design & Layout
Meerkat Graphics, Inc.
Lolo, Montana

Published in the U.S.A. by
Phoenix Publishing Co.
P.O. Box 8231
Missoula, Montana 59807

INTRODUCTION

When I was a child of four or five my favorite storybook was Doctor Dan the Band Aid Man. It was the story of a boy who fixes his friends when they feel sick or are bleeding. I knew even then that was what I wanted to do when I grew up.

As a child of eight or nine I loved to read mystery books like Nancy Drew and The Hardy Boys. I was intrigued with the clues that seemed meaningless until Nancy Drew placed them in the context of the mystery question and organized them into an amazing solution that at the end seemed all too obvious. I dreamt of being an investigator when I grew up.

I am now grown. I have been a physical therapist for over 30 years and I have been writing books on health and medicine for five years. As I was pondering the content for an introduction to this latest book, it came to me that incontinence has been the mystery I've been trying to solve for the past ten years in clinical practice. I have been collecting the clues from widely diverse locations, placing them in the context of the mystery question, and organizing them into an "amazing" solution that "fixes" individuals who are "sick" or have a disabling condition. I am really doing what I dreamt of as a child.

Incontinence has been a mystery to men and women, especially as they age. Loss of bladder control is not talked about in public or private, creating a shroud of mystery. In the not too distant past physicians did not always ask questions about incontinence during a history and physical examination. Men and women still only tell the physician about incontinence problems half the time. Without communication of facts the mystery of incontinence and its treatment grows.

The mystery of effective incontinence treatment in the elderly has had several disparate clues. Physicians have treatment clues of medication and surgery to treat incontinence. Nurses have treatment clues of bladder training, prompted voiding, and assisted voiding. Physical therapists have treatment clues of pelvic muscle exercises and physiological quieting. Occupational therapists have treatment clues for life style changes, adaptive clothing and devices. Generally these clues have been held in secret places for the exclusive use of the professionals to dispense. It has been rare that any one individual persevered as a detective to sleuth out all of the clues in the various medical professions. Furthermore, even when all of the clues have been collected, the job of organizing them into an effective "fix" for the incontinence problem has been even more remote.

The purpose of this book is to bring together the disparate clues of the incontinence treatment mystery by organizing the clues in the context of the mystery, and to solve the mystery of incontinence for each individual in a seemingly simple solution. Just because incontinence is a mystery doesn't mean it cannot have an easy, effective solution. The solution has been complicated because the clues were so widely dispersed and unorganized. This book brings the clues together to solve the mystery. It describes a behavioral and exercise approach to the treatment of incontinence in a variety of populations including the active or frail elderly, the elderly living independently or in nursing homes, and the cognitively aware or the elderly with dementia. The purpose of this book is to prevent and/or treat the incontinence that becomes more prevalent as we age through education, life style changes, and exercise.

A medical consult is essential before beginning a program to treat incontinence. A medical assessment can pinpoint the possible reasons for the incontinence and direct the treatment.

This book is designed for the reader to follow the basic Chapters 1-8 before finding the chapter(s) on the appropriate patient group he/she is interested in (Chapters 9-13).

TABLE OF CONTENTS

Chapter 1	Common Myths and Mysteries	1
Chapter 2	Anatomy/Physiology for the Clinican and Client	7
Chapter 3	Types and Causes of Urinary Incontinence	17
Chapter 4	Fecal Incontinence/Constipation	23
Chapter 5	Beyond Kegels Exercises and Physiological Quieting	30
Chapter 6	Biofeedback: How Can it Help with Exercises for Incontinence?	59
Chapter 7	Life Style Changes for Continence	63
Chapter 8	What Medications Can Help?	74
Chapter 9	Confident and Continent Prevention Program	81
Chapter 10	The Active Elderly at Home and Independent	85
Chapter 11	The Frail Elderly	102
Chapter 12	Total Hip Replacement, Hip Fracture, and Incontinence	142
Chapter 13	For Men Only	150
Chapter 14	Protective Products for Incontinence	162
Resources		165
References		168
Glossary		171

CHAPTER 1

COMMON MYTHS AND MYSTERIES

The many myths about incontinence lead elderly to have many questions that go unanswered and untreated. The lack of understanding and lack of treatment leads to decreased independence and self worth. This chapter gives a brief look at what the facts and fiction are and how they relate to the elderly.

Incontinence, in anyone over 60, has a significant impact on their well being and independence. When the elderly have an incontinence problem it affects their independence because shame and fear often keep them isolated at home instead of going out to socialize with friends. Furthermore, when they do go outside the home it limits their activities because the availability of an accessible toilet becomes paramount. The need for assistance and external devices for bladder and bowel control decreases independence and may create the need to transfer to a more restrictive, unfamiliar environment. The cost of pads, assistive devices, and disposal of pads can use dollars that would otherwise be available for food, rent, medications, or outside socialization.

Physical and emotional well-being is impacted with incontinence. Incontinence leads to decreased physical activity as the individual attempts to prevent leaking. Muscle weakness and atrophy, joint stiffness, and decreased physical endurance occur secondary to the decreased physical activity. Incontinence increases the risk of falls when the individual tries to hurry to the bathroom. There is an increased frequency of bladder and vaginal infections with incontinence. In the frail elderly incontinence increases the frequency of decubiti/bed sores and interferes with their healing.

The impact of all these factors in the elderly is a decrease in self esteem and feelings of self efficacy (personal control). Depression related to incontinence often ensues, impacting feelings of well-being and self worth. Incontinence is the second most common reason the elderly enter the nursing home environment.

The multiple factors associated with incontinence leave those involved with many questions. The questions elderly individuals often ask about incontinence include:
1. Is urinary incontinence a normal part of aging and not preventable?
2. What can I do about it? How can I keep from getting worse?
3. How can I minimize its interference in my active life?
4. Why didn't the surgery I had fix the problem for good?
5. Why do my bladder and bowel quit working before

my brain, heart, or lungs?

The questions often asked by health care professionals include:
1. Is urinary incontinence an inevitable part of aging and not fixable?
2. If it is not part of normal aging, what causes it?
3. Is effective treatment available?
4. Does knowing the cause change the treatment?
5. What is the minimum information needed to plan treatment?

The common mysteries about urinary incontinence (UI) in the aging population include:

1. UI is normal with aging.

In fact, while UI is more common with age, it is not inevitable. Approximately eighty percent of elderly individuals have changes in bladder physiology, but not all of those have incontinence. Fifty to sixty percent of elderly individuals experience UI in some form at some time in their life.

2. UI is inevitable in demented elderly.

The fact is, incontinence increases with dementia, but in the early stages of dementia and Alzheimers most individuals can be continent. Approximately half of the individuals with severe dementia or Alzheimers have incontinence problems. Being bed-bound increases incontinence significantly.

3. UI in nursing homes is inevitable because of drugs and disease.

UI is never inevitable, even if mental ability and mobility are decreased. Even some bed-bound individuals can be continent with assistance. Diseases and drugs are not the only causes of incontinence. Consider each resident's function and his/her capabilities. Risk factors aside from disease and drugs for UI in nursing homes include:
1. Dependent transfers.
2. Dependent dressing.
3. Vision impairment.
4. Hearing impairment.
5. Manual dexterity.
6. Range of motion limitations.

4. The major cause of incontinence in nursing homes is detrusor instability and is not treatable.

Fifty to sixty percent of nursing home incontinence is due to abnormal detrusor (bladder) activity. Forty to fifty percent is due to either bladder obstruction such as prostate enlargement in men, functional limitations, or pelvic muscle dysfunction in men and women.

In reality, detrusor instability, bladder obstruction, pelvic muscle dysfunction, and functional limitations are all treatable.

5. The cause of the UI will determine the treatment.

In fact, there are multiple causes of UI. It is equally important to assess the dysfunction and life style

compensatory mechanisms in each individual as it is to determine treatment. Compensatory mechanisms can include:
1. Decreasing fluid intake.
2. Increasing voiding frequency.
3. Identifying all toilet locations.
4. Altering dress.
5. Limiting social experiences.

Treating life style compensatory mechanisms and considering transient/acute and functional/environmental causes of UI will determine the next level of treatment.

The following chapters will discuss:
1. The anatomy and function of the urogenital and pelvic muscle systems as they relate to urinary continence.
2. The types of urinary incontinence.
3. The effect of fecal incontinence on the urinary system.
4. Exercise and behavioral treatment to maintain or improve continence in subpopulations of the elderly.
5. Protective products to enable an active, full life style.

PELVIC MUSCLE FORCE FIELD

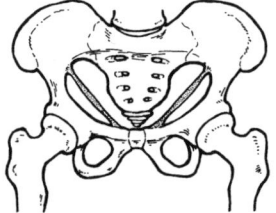

**Obturator Tendon/
Arcuate Tendon**
Figure 2-1

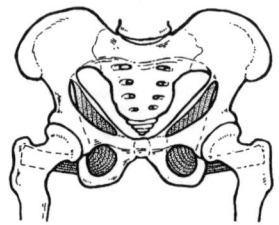

Obturator Internus
Figure 2-2

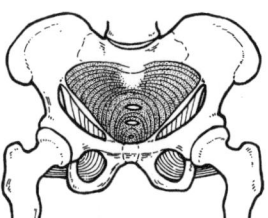

**Pelvic Diaphragm/
Levator Ani**
Figure 2-3

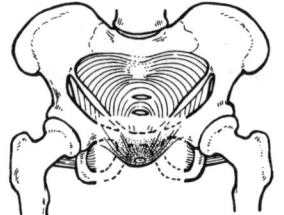

**Urogenital Diaphragm/
Perineum**
Figure 2-4

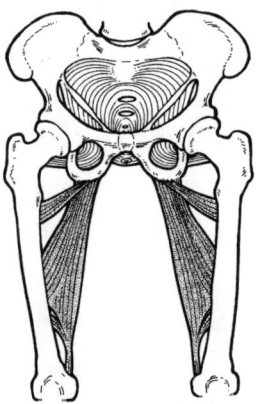

Adductors
Figure 2-5

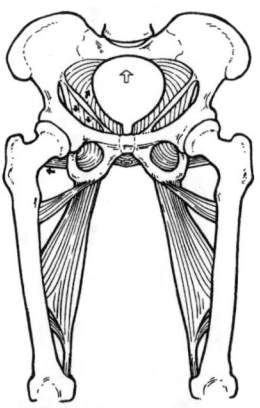

**Bladder Support
Muscle Force Field**
Figure 2-6

CHAPTER 2

ANATOMY/PHYSIOLOGY FOR THE CLINICIAN AND CLIENT

FOR THE CLINICIAN

THE MUSCLES OF CONTINENCE
Striated Muscles

Striated muscles are innervated by the voluntary nervous system.

The **obturator internus** attaches externally to the greater trochanter of the femur, travels through the lesser sciatic notch of the pelvis at a 120° angle, and attaches inside the pelvis on the arcuate tendon and around the obturator foramen (Fig. 2-2).

The **pelvic diaphragm/levator ani** attaches to the arcuate tendon and to anterior, posterior, and lateral aspects of the lower pelvis and sacrum (Fig. 2-3).

The **urogenital diaphragm/perineum** attaches to the symphysis pubis, pubic rami, the perineal body, and ischial tuberosities. It interdigitates via fascia and connective tissue with the pelvic diaphragm (Fig. 2-4).

The **external sphincter** is imbedded in the urogenital diaphragm muscles and interdigitates with the pelvic diaphragm muscle.

The **adductor muscles** attach to the medial aspect of the femur and to the pubic rami adjacent to the urogenital diaphragm attachment (Fig. 2-5).

Smooth Muscles

The smooth muscles are innervated by the autonomic nervous system.

The **detrusor (bladder)** is composed of three layers of circular and longitudinal muscles (Fig. 2-6). The trigone area at the base of the bladder is the location of entry for the ureters.

The **urethra** connects with the bladder at the bladder neck. It contains longitudinal and circular smooth muscle layers that contract to maintain continence.

LIGAMENTS AND FASCIA OF CONTINENCE

The **obturator/arcuate tendon** runs from front to back in the lower pelvis bilaterally (Fig. 2-1). The obturator internus and pelvic diaphragm muscles attach to it. The urethropelvic ligament and periurethral fascia blend with it.

The **urethropelvic ligament** stabilizes the urethra and blends with the obturator tendon to provide support to the bladder neck and proximal urethra. (The periurethral and endopelvic fascia are a continuation of the ligamentous support surrounding the urethra, vagina, and cervix of the uterus.)

The **pubourethral ligament** attaches to the symphysis pubis and fascia to support and stabilize the mid-urethra.

In the urogenital area ligaments and fascia have contractile capability, i.e. there is contractile tissue intermingled with connective, noncontractile tissue.

CONTINENCE AND THE PELVIC MUSCLES

The pelvic muscle support of the internal organs (bladder, uterus and bowel) and continence involves:
1. Skeletal attachments for stability on the lower pelvis, sacrum, coccyx, and femur.
2. Ligamentous and fascial interconnectedness and interdigitation with striated muscle for stability and force transfer.
3. A pulley system of organ suspension combining the obturator internus attachment to the arcuate tendon to the pelvic diaphragm (levator ani) which is interconnected with the urogenital diaphragm (perineum) and external sphincter muscle groups. A bilateral contraction of the obturator internus muscles effectively lifts the "hammock" that supports the organs within the pelvis and closes the urethra. A bilateral contraction of the adductors relengthens the obturators and facilitates urogenital and pelvic diaphragm contraction.
4. Autonomic and voluntary nervous system integration to coordinate the contraction and function of smooth muscle (bladder, uterus, and bowel) with striated muscle (pelvic and urogenital diaphragm).

Continence is maintained by optimal bladder and bowel position, appropriate intra-abdominal pressure forces, effective muscle action and integrated reflex responses.

The pelvic muscle support for continence can be pictured as an old fashioned clothesline with (Fig. 2-7):
1. A post at each end (the sacrum and symphysis pubis).

2. Two clothes lines (arcuate tendons).
3. A hammock hung between the two clotheslines (pelvic diaphragm).
4. The ground (greater trochanter of the femur).
5. Tethers attached laterally to the clothes line and the ground (obturator internus).
6. The peach basket (urogenital diaphragm and external sphincter).

The lower pelvis, sacrum, and coccyx are attachments for the arcuate tendons and pelvic muscles. The hammock (pelvic diaphragm) attaches to lateral pelvis, sacrum, symphysis pubis, and arcuate tendons. The tethers (obturator internus) attach to the clothesline (arcuate tendon) and the ground (greater trochanter of the femur) through a pulley system (the lesser sciatic notch). The

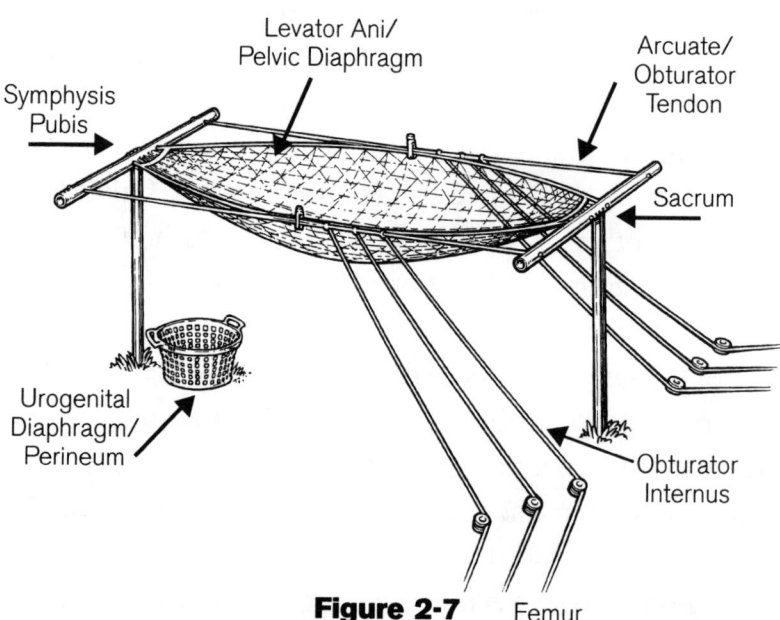

Figure 2-7

peach basket (urogenital diaphragm and external sphincter) interdigitates with the hammock (pelvic diaphragm) and sits in the front 1/3-1/2 of the perineal area.

As the tethers (obturator internus) tighten they pull the clotheslines laterally which lifts the hammock (pelvic diaphragm) up and out.

As the hammock (pelvic diaphragm) lifts up and out it elevates the bladder, uterus, and bowel. This maintains the optimum bladder-urethral angle and anorectal angle for continence. It facilitates the sphincteric action and coaptation (approximation of) walls of the urethra for continence. It maintains the bladder-urethral pressure gradient for continence.

As the hammock (pelvic diaphragm) lifts up and out it also facilitates optimal positioning and closure of the bottom of the peach basket (urogenital diaphragm and external sphincter).

This muscular force field is the primary support for the pelvic organs. The tendons, ligaments, and fasciae are all secondary in that if a defect in the muscular support occurs the tendon/ligament/fascial support will be unable to maintain organ position on its own.

NEUROLOGY OF CONTINENCE

The **voluntary nervous system** (VNS), from **sacral nerve roots two, three, and four** sends and receives information from the pelvic and urogenital diaphragm and external sphincter muscles via the **pudendal nerve.** The voluntary nervous system, from sacral nerve roots two, three, and four via the pelvic nerve, innervates the obturator internus.

The Voluntary Nervous System

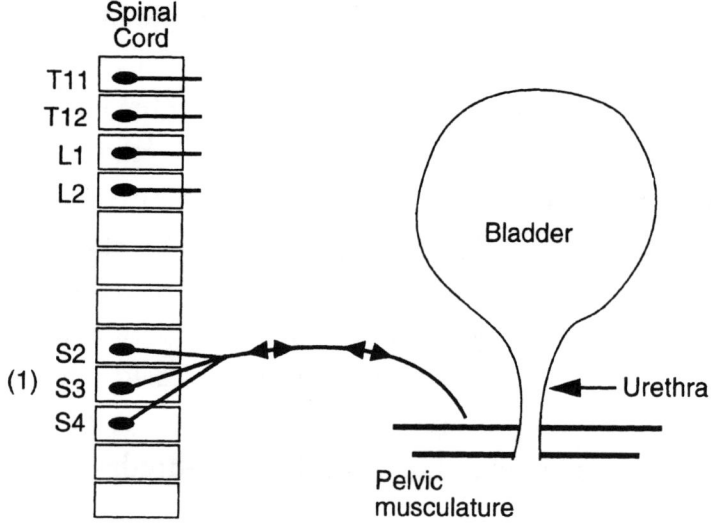

Figure 2-8

The Autonomic Nervous System

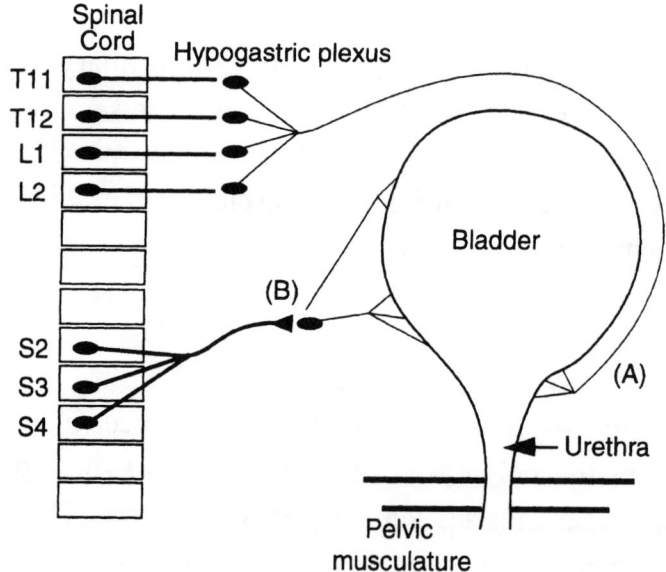

Figure 2-9 A & B

The **autonomic nervous system** (ANS) innervates the bladder, urethra, bowel, and rectum. There are three parts of the autonomic nervous system:

The **sympathetic system**
Hypogastric plexus – nerve roots Thoracic 10, 11, 12, Lumbar 1, 2. Innervates primarily bladder neck and proximal urethra (Fig. 2-9 A).

The **parasympathetic system**
Pelvic plexus – nerve roots Sacral 2, 3, 4.
Innervates primarily bladder wall (Fig. 2-9 B).

The **enteric system**
Innervates the gut from esophagus to anus.

The voluntary and autonomic nervous systems work together to maintain continence. Toileting activities occur less than one hour each day. For over 23 hours of the day:

The pelvic diaphragm is maintaining a resting tone adequate to position and help maintain the bladder neck/proximal urethra closed. A striated muscle's resting tone is largely determined by the autonomic nervous system. The gamma bias of the muscle spindle is "set" by the ANS.

The detrusor muscle is maintaining a resting tone adequate to allow expansion of bladder size without setting off detrusor contractions (largely inhibition of smooth muscle contraction is controlled by the autonomic nervous system).

When the urge to urinate or have a bowel movement is perceived in the brain, the voluntary nervous system comes into play more:

The pelvic diaphragm and external sphincters contract volitionally.

This contraction via a spinal reflex arc, inhibits the detrusor muscle contractions until urination is appropriate or inhibits the rectum and anus until defecation is appropriate.

This interaction implies that afferent messages from the voluntary nervous system travel to the spinal cord and synapse with autonomic efferent fibers to transmit inhibitory messages to the bladder wall.

When it is appropriate to urinate or have a bowel movement the VNS and ANS coordinate so:

The pelvic muscles relax and,

The bladder (detrusor muscle) contracts to empty the bladder of urine.

In bowel function the pelvic muscles relax and the smooth muscle of the rectum and anus contract to empty the stool.

There are as many as 16 reflex arcs between bowel, bladder, spinal cord and brain, all of which control continence.

From birth until approximately three years of age, elimination is primarily controlled via the pons. At approximately three, when a child can count to ten, the cortex becomes dominant in elimination control and potty training is successful. Until then the caretaker is trained more than the child. In the elderly, as cognitive function declines the cortex releases primary control and once again the pons becomes more dominant in elimination. Pons control is an unconscious process. When the afferent messages of bladder stretching are received, the efferent message is to pause, release the pelvic muscles, and push to eliminate the urine or feces without concern for time or place. It is important to stimulate the cortex to keep it as an active director of bladder and bowel control in the elderly.

The **enteric nervous system** is known as the gut's brain. It is located in tissue lining the esophagus, stomach, small and large intestine, and colon. The enteric nervous system can function alone, separate from the central nervous system with its network of electrical and chemical messengers. It can also act interdependently with the head brain via the vagus nerve.

The gut contains 100 million neurons – even more than the spinal cord. It is composed of complex integrated circuits and blood brain barriers, much like the head brain. "Gut Feelings" determine happiness and misery to a large extent. Abdominal pain, difficulty swallowing, and bowel problems are from the brain of the gut, more often than the brain in the head. Neurotransmitters in the gut brain include: serotonin, dopamine, norepinephrine, noradrenaline, nitric oxide, enkephalins, benzodiazepines, neuropeptides, and immune system cells.

When the enertic nervous system of the gut is dysfunctional, transit time of food through the intestines is affected. This can result in constipation, diarrhea, and/or pain. Any dysfunction in the intestine often leads to bladder dysfunction.

The following pages are an easy, illustrated explanation of striated muscle function in bladder control.

FOR THE CLIENT
MUSCLES THAT AID IN BLADDER CONTROL – HOW THEY WORK

Your bladder is like a balloon sitting in a hammock.

The position of the hammock can keep you dry ...

or allow leaking.

When your hammock muscle is lifted it prevents leaking. The bladder outlet is closed to keep you dry.

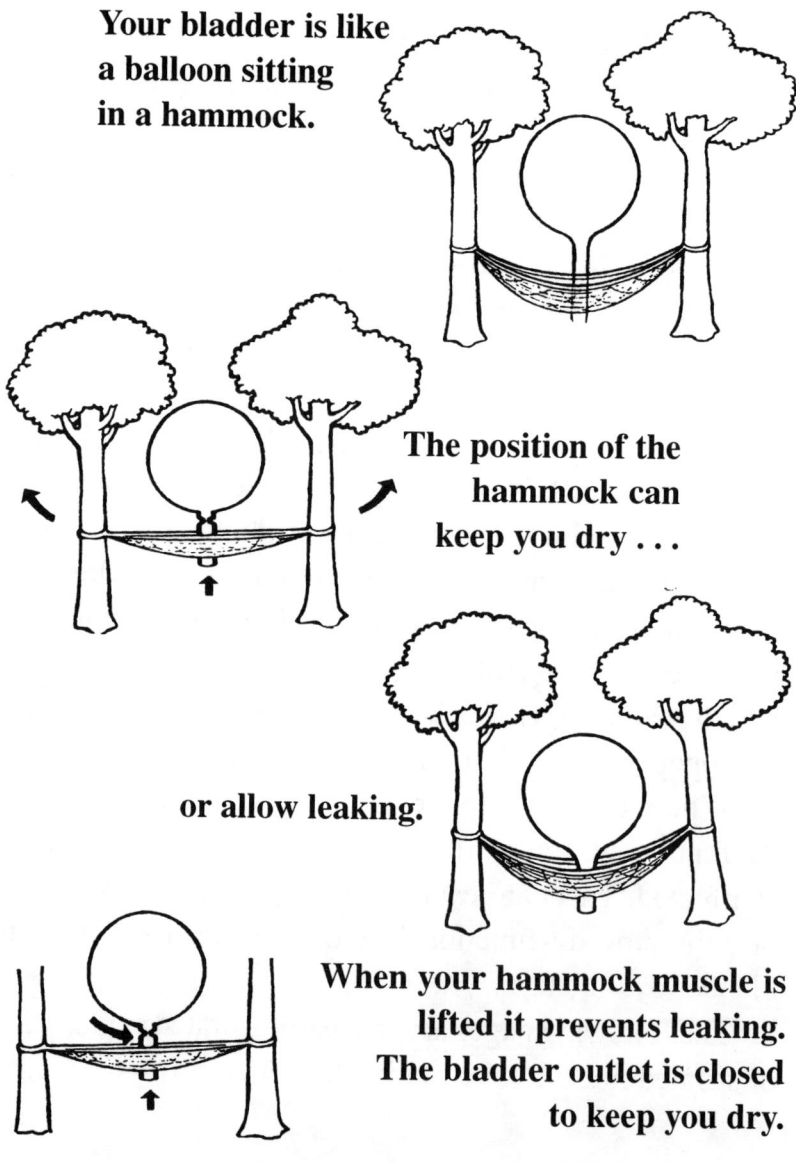

CHAPTER 3

TYPES AND CAUSES OF URINARY INCONTINENCE

ACUTE/TRANSIENT INCONTINENCE
PERSISTENT/CHRONIC INCONTINENCE

Urinary incontinence can be divided into two general categories – transient and chronic.

ACUTE/TRANSIENT INCONTINENCE
Transient incontinence implies that the individual is normally continent, however because of an acute illness, infection, etc. there is involuntary loss of urine. If the problem of illness or infection is treated the incontinence is eliminated.

Urinary Tract Infection (UTI)
Dysuria, painful urination, and urgency as a result of UTI, may defeat the ability to reach the toilet in time.

Atrophic Urethritis or Vaginitis (Hypoestrogenism)
Hypoestrogenism (decreased estrogen) causes atrophic

changes in genitourinary and pelvic muscle systems. Dysuria, dyspareunia (painful intercourse), burning during urination, and urgency are common symptoms.

Stool impaction

Bowel dysfunction leads to urge and stress bladder incontinence. Any bowel problem affects the urinary system due to the proximity and shared nerve innervation.

Diuretics

The bladder is overwhelmed with fluid leading to polyuria, frequency, and urge incontinence. Diuretics may increase the severity of already present incontinence.

Caffeine

Caffeine acts as a diuretic. It is also a bladder muscle irritant and a nervous system irritant. Frequency and urge incontinence often occur.

Other Medications

Anticholinergic agents such as Ditropan or Levsin, medications often used for gastrointestinal motor disorder, Parkinson's Disease or heart dysrhythmias, can lead to urinary retention, frequency, overflow, and/or functional incontinence.

Sedatives, hypnotics, CNS depressants, and alcohol accumulate in the elderly and can cause confusion and impaired mobility leading to secondary incontinence and/or functional incontinence.

Alpha-adrenergic agents such as antihistamines and

sympathomimetics (decongestants) can induce retention and overflow incontinence.

Calcium channel blockers reduce smooth muscle contractility causing retention and overflow incontinence.

Delirium

Incontinence is often an associated symptom to delirium.

Psychological

The relationship between psychological conditions and incontinence is not completely understood but is documented.

Restricted Mobility

Limited mobility secondary to a chronic illness or injury (arthritis, poor eyesight, Parkinson's disease, stroke) can lead to functional incontinence.

Increased Urine Production

Hyperglycemia and hypercalcemia can lead to excessive fluid intake followed by diuresis and incontinence. Excessive fluid intake or volume overload from venous insufficiency with edema or congestive heart failure can lead to incontinence.

PERSISTENT/CHRONIC INCONTINENCE

Chronic incontinence implies the individual has lost urinary control for at least six months in relation to physical activity, overactive bladder contractions, dysfunctional pelvic muscle function, neurological impairment, and/or dementia. Subcategories of chronic incontinence include:

Stress Incontinence

The individual is unable to hold urine when intra-abdominal pressure increases. This may be caused by an underactive urethra, decreased bladder outlet resistance, an unstable urethra, or genuine stress incontinence (GSI). In females, decreased pelvic muscle tone and/or estrogen depletion leading to atrophic vaginitis/urethritis can lead to stress incontinence. In males, urethral damage following radical prostatectomy and reduced urethral closure pressure from medication use (alpha adrenergic blockers for hypertension) are the most common causes.

The individual presents with loss of urine when coughing, sneezing, laughing, getting up from sitting or lying down, bending, pushing, or pulling.

Urge Incontinence

The individual is unable to inhibit voiding when the sensation to void is present. This may be caused by detrusor (bladder) instability, hyperreflexia, overactive, uninhibited or unstable bladder. In males and females causes include bladder tumors or stones, high volume voids secondary to diuretics or excessive intake, urinary tract infection, inflammation, radiation therapy, concentrated urine, or limited functional bladder capacity. In females estrogen deficiency leading to atrophic vaginitis/urethritis may cause urge incontinence.

The individual presents with the awareness of an urgent

need to void but not enough lead time to get to the toilet.

Mixed Incontinence
The individual experiences a combination of stress and urge incontinence with symptoms of both.

Overflow Incontinence (Retention)
The individual is unable to completely empty the bladder when voiding. This may be caused by an atonic, flaccid, neuropathic, paralytic, or underactive bladder. Possible causes include decreased bladder contractility, neurologic disease, surgery, pharmacotherapy (anticholinergics, psychotropics, anti-parkinsonians, antispasmodics, opiates, Beta adrenergic blockers) or chronic overdistention of the bladder. Other causes may be urethral obstruction from stricture, enlarged prostate, cystocele, or stool impaction. Increased sphincteric resistance from pharmacotherapy (antihistamines, alpha adrenergic stimulants) or obstructive atrophic vaginitis/urethritis (from postmenopausal estrogen deficiency) can cause retention and overflow.

The individual presents with toileting frequently in small amounts and may be continent or incontinent.

Reflex Incontinence
The individual is unable to inhibit voiding because sensation is absent. Possible causes include diseases, injuries, or neurologic disorders interfering with communication between the brain and bladder; delirium or medications may be implicated (analgesics or

tranquilizers); CVA; dementia; demyelinating diseases; peripheral nerve lesions; trauma; and severe mental retardation.

The individual presents with loss of urine but no awareness of the leaking.

Continuous Incontinence

The individual is unable to hold any urine. The individual presents with constant dribbling of urine. Possible causes include structural damage to the urethra post surgery, post radical prostatectomy, hysterectomy, and/or bladder augmentation.

Environmental/Functional Incontinence

The individual is physically unable to get to or use the toilet. It is a functional problem. Often there is more attention paid to protecting the environment from urine rather than using the environment to promote continence. Environmental or functional incontinence may be caused by confusion or disorientation (medications such as sedatives or hypnotics may be implicated), an unfamiliar environment, inaccessible or inadequate facilities, visual disturbances (impairing ability to see the toilet), physical disabilities or mechanical barriers (preventing full, independent mobility), inaccessible clothing, pain, or lack of security or privacy.

The individual presents with an awareness of the need to void (without urgency), but can't get to or use the toilet.

CHAPTER 4

FECAL INCONTINENCE/ CONSTIPATION

Fecal incontinence is the involuntary loss of gas, liquid, or solid stool. Constipation and/or diarrhea affect urinary incontinence because of the proximity of the organ structures in the pelvis and the similar neurological innervation. It is reported that fecal incontinence is as high as fifty percent in nursing homes. The high incidence of fecal problems in the elderly, especially those in nursing homes, contributes to higher levels of bladder incontinence. It is therefore important to address bowel habits during the initial assessment and treatment of urinary incontinence. Assessment includes a medical and surgical history, a bowel diary, a medication history, and physical exam.

The elderly are often obsessed with their bowel function. Many use laxatives regularly, and in nursing homes enemas are often a frequent remedy. These practices alone can cause problems, eventually damaging colonic activity and nerve transmission.

The gastrointestinal (GI) tract is a tube within a tube, one tube of circular muscle, the other of longitudinal muscle that propel the bolus of food through the tract from mouth to anus. The tubes are primarily innervated by the enteric nervous system, a subdivision of the autonomic nervous system.

In the elderly there is decreased motility (prolonged transit time) due to atrophy of smooth muscle and mucosa and impaired enteric nervous system function. The motility can be affected in one portion of the GI tract more than another. When colon transit time is prolonged excessive fluid is reabsorbed and the bolus becomes hard and difficult to pass. The individual often describes pain in the right upper abdominal quadrant but on palpation tenderness is difficult to find.

Constipation can be caused by a nonrelaxing puborectalis muscle. The puborectalis muscle, a portion of the levator ani muscle group, forms a sling that maintains the anorectal angle until it is time to have a bowel movement. At that time the puborectalis muscle must release, decreasing the anorectal angle, which allows the feces to move down the rectum and out the anus. If the puborectalis fails to relax, the feces remains in the rectum and descending colon during pushing. It becomes hard and compacted, i.e. constipating.

Decreased frequency of bowel movements is normal with age and not necessarily an indication of constipation. Two or fewer bowel movements per week are considered abnormal. If bowel movements are less frequent and/or hard or difficult to pass then constipation is often an appropriate label.

Fecal impaction is one of the most common causes of

fecal and urinary incontinence, especially in the elderly. Chronic constipation results in absorption of the fluid content of the feces leading to hard, rocklike stools in the bowel. Mucous and bacteria develop around the hard stool producing a foul-smelling brown liquid that is excreted as a diarrhea-like substance. Colorectal surgeons refer to it as pseudoincontinence. The liquid stool may be continuous and uncontrollable. If the individual is treated for diarrhea the problem is only aggravated. Correct diagnosis can be done through digital rectal palpation and abdominal x-ray.

When there is a correct diagnosis of constipation and/or impaction, treatment to clear the impaction is primary. This is usually achieved through medication and/or an enema. For example, colace liquid added to an enema can help soften the impaction making the break up easier. It is then important to prevent the reoccurrence of the problem. Alterations in diet, exercise, and pelvic muscle function are effective methods of treatment.

Many men after radical prostatectomy may have bowel concerns. The tissue between the rectum and the remaining urethra is thin and fragile so pressure of a very hard stool or strong pushing can cause bleeding from the surgical site. For at least three months after surgery the area is vulnerable. During this time constipation is more common due to pain medications, inactivity, possible dehydration, and dietary changes. Since enemas can be dangerous to the integrity of the rectal tissue stool softeners are used in addition to diet, exercise, and fluid intake.

Individuals with heart conditions will often have bowel concerns. Straining with constipation after a heart attack can lead to vagal nerve reaction and a possible second myocardial infarction thus it is imperative to keep the stools soft and to keep a regular schedule of bowel movements. Dietary changes, a regular bowel protocol, stool softeners, or laxatives are helpful.

For the elderly, a bowel program is indicated when one of the following occurs:
1. Bowel movements are two or fewer a week.
2. There is fecal staining of underwear.
3. Medications or enemas are used for bowel movements.
4. There is straining and or pain in attempting a bowel movement.
5. There is the feeling of incomplete bowel emptying.

The goals of the bowel program are to:
1. Increase frequency of normal bowel movements to greater than two times of week.
2. Eliminate fecal soiling, constipation, and diarrhea.
3. Decrease or eliminate the need for enemas or medication.
4. Eliminate straining and/or pain while attempting a bowel movement.
5. Increase daily activities without bowel incontinence interference.

To accomplish these goals four major areas must be addressed:
1. Nutrition.

2. Bowel habit protocol.
3. Exercise.
4. Diaphragmatic breathing.

Nutritional recommendations for healthy bowel movements include:
1. Six to eight glasses of noncaffeinated fluid daily.
2. Five servings of cooked or raw fruits and vegetables per day: one at breakfast, two at lunch, two at dinner. Vegetables should be raw or lightly cooked to retain the roughage and nutritional qualities. Prunes, figs, apricots, oranges, and grapefruit are fruits with laxative qualities.
3. Bran and yogurt at breakfast, 1-3 teaspoons unrefined wheat bran or 1 tablespoon flaxseed (ground) sprinkled on 4-6 ounces of yogurt with fresh fruit is a good combination. The bran or flaxseed provides the roughage, while the yogurt is high in calcium and easy to swallow. Another combination includes 2 cups applesauce, 1 cup prune juice, and 1/2 cup bran. Use it on toast or eat 1-3 tablespoons a day.
4. An additional consideration is a vitamin/mineral supplement of 250-500mg magnesium and/or 250-2000mg of vitamin C with physician approval. Magnesium is a smooth muscle relaxant that helps to relax the GI tract. Vitamin C is essential for GI health, however too much causes diarrhea so increase vitamin C to the amount just before diarrhea.

A daily **bowel habit protocol** includes morning massage, fluid intake, and daily toilet time. Before arising in the morning the individual performs gentle abdominal self massage. The instructions are: " using the fingertips trace clockwise circles starting at the lower right abdomen, going up then across at the bellybutton level and down the left side. Repeat the sequence three times. After arising drink 1-2 cups of warm water 30 minutes before breakfast. This technique stimulates colonic activity. After breakfast sit on the toilet for 5-7 minutes in a comfortable position with feet well supported on the floor or a footstool, hips and knees at approximately 90° of flexion, knees slightly higher than hips. Practice diaphragmatic breathing. Relax the pelvic muscles by rolling the knees in and out 3-4 times, then releasing the muscles completely. If there is a problem with straining to have a bowel movement, the individual needs to inhale and exhale in short staccatos as if blowing bubbles while pushing.

A **daily exercise program** is essential for bowel health. The two components of exercise include:
1. Pelvic muscle exercises. Beyond Kegels–Easy, Active–roll in and roll out exercises done in bed before arising and before going to sleep at night (see p. 33).
2. Moderate aerobic exercise for 20-30 minutes daily. Walking is preferred because of its affect on the pelvic and bowel muscles. Biking and swimming are other options.

A **daily diaphragmatic breathing routine** is effective in optimizing the bowel function. Practicing for 3-5 minutes 2-3 times/day can have a significant effect on bowel health (see p. 55).

When conservative measures have been tried and additional intervention is needed medications, suppositories, or enemas are available. Options include over the counter magnesium citrate liquid, mineral oil, and stool softeners. Prescription medications such as cisapride (Propulsid) 5-20mg 15-30 minutes before a meal can improve colon health and decrease constipation when there is prolonged transit time in all or in a portion of the GI tract and when a diagnosis of gastrointestinal motor disorder has been determined. Metoclopromide (Reglan) is another medication that can be helpful in improving transit time.

All supplements, suppositories, and other interventions need to be discussed with the physician. Bowel function can be a positive influence on urinary continence patterns if the functional changes of aging are understood and treated appropriately.

CHAPTER 5

BEYOND KEGELS EXERCISES AND PHYSIOLOGICAL QUIETING

BEYOND KEGELS EXERCISES

The Beyond Kegels exercises are designed to develop the pelvic muscle force field that supports the bladder, uterus, and bowel. The pelvic muscle force field consists of the obturator internus, pelvic diaphragm, urogenital diaphragm, sphincters, and adductors. The Beyond Kegels exercises develop the strength, coordination, and work-rest capability of the pelvic muscle force field. As the legs roll in and out, the pelvic diaphragm is maintained in a relatively stable position, facilitated by the obturator internus and adductors. In this way the bladder and urethra are maintained in an optimal position while the pelvic diaphragm goes through its rest/work cycle. The bladder outlet/urethra is maintained in a closed position until the pelvic diaphragm is consciously released to urinate.

The easiest Beyond Kegels exercises can be done by even the most frail or confused elderly individual. The Beyond Kegels–Easy, Active Exercises can be done in bed or in a chair. The Roll Out exercise activates the obturator internus muscles. The Roll In exercise activates the adductor muscles. When these become easy, Beyond Kegels – Easy, Resistive Exercises can be added using a Kegelband and Kegelball. It is not necessary for the individual to focus on or actively tighten the pelvic diaphragm/levator ani in these first two phases of Beyond Kegels Exercises.

The more advanced Beyond Kegels Exercises – Active, Resistive combine active contraction of the obturators and adductors with the pelvic and urogenital diaphragm muscles. The individual contracts the pelvic diaphragm as the legs roll out or roll in.

Standing Plíe exercises activate the pelvic muscle force field in the standing position. The easiest level of this exercise is to simply bend the knees 1-2" slowly and return slowly to standing. The knee bends are done with the feet pointing out. The next level of difficulty for the Standing Plíe is to lift the pelvic diaphragm simultaneously with the knees bending and straightening.

Quick Contractions of the urogenital diaphragm and sphincter muscles strengthen and improve the response time of these muscles for reflex protection with coughing, sneezing, etc.

In addition to the Beyond Kegels exercises, breathing and quieting unwanted muscle activity is important. That is accomplished with Physiological Quieting (PQ) activities. PQ includes diaphragmatic breathing and hand warming as well as body/mind quieting.

The length and duration of an exercise session varies with the ability of the individual. If someone is very weak or debilitated from surgery, radiation, or chemotherapy, or has a neurological condition that creates fatigue, a short duration of exercise 2-4 times a day is recommended. For the frail elderly, 10 repetitions 2-3 times a day may be sufficient. A gradual increase in time and repetitions over several weeks is usually tolerated well.

In general, for the active elderly the exercise session duration recommended is:

First Week:	3-5 minutes, 3 times a day
Second Week:	5-7 minutes, 3-5 times a day
Third Week:	7-10 minutes, 2 times a day
Fourth Week:	10 minutes, 2 times a day

An exercise session begins and ends with 30-60 seconds of Relaxed Awareness of pelvic muscles, several slow diaphragmatic breaths, and release head to toe into the support of chair or bed. It progresses to Roll In, Roll Out exercises emphasizing equal work and rest periods for 2-6 minutes. Standing Plíe and/or Quick Contract and Release exercises are included when appropriate. Ten repetitions of each is adequate. Other exercises are added as deemed necessary. Physiological Quieting is practiced 20 minutes nightly using the audiotape. Diaphragmatic breathing and hand warming are practiced hourly for 30-60 seconds if urge is present.

BEYOND KEGELS – EASY, ACTIVE EXERCISES

To lift your hammock muscle roll your knees apart then bring them back together. This helps strengthen the hammock muscle and prevent leaking.

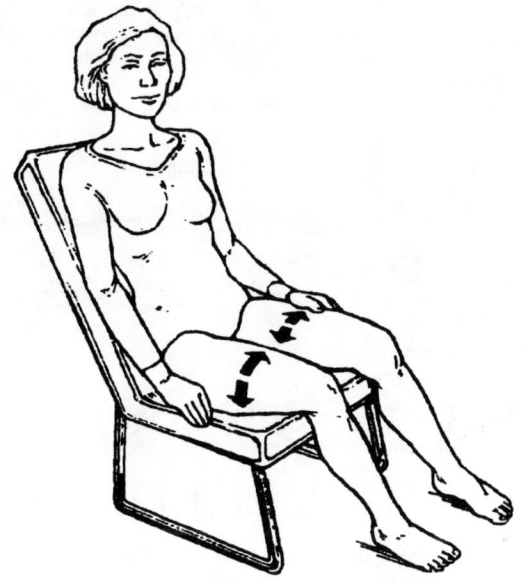

Every morning, middle of the day, and evening do the exercise of rolling or pushing your knees out and then bringing them back in – 10 repetitions. You can do the exercise either in a sitting position or lying down.

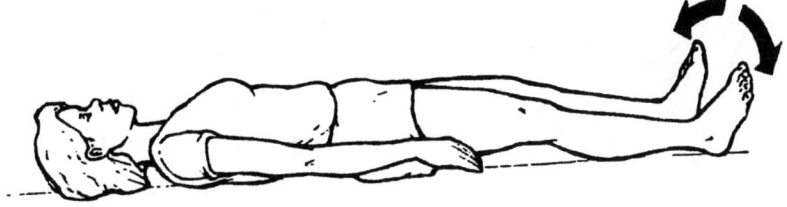

BEYOND KEGELS – EASY, RESISTIVE EXERCISES

When the exercises become easy you can add some resistance.

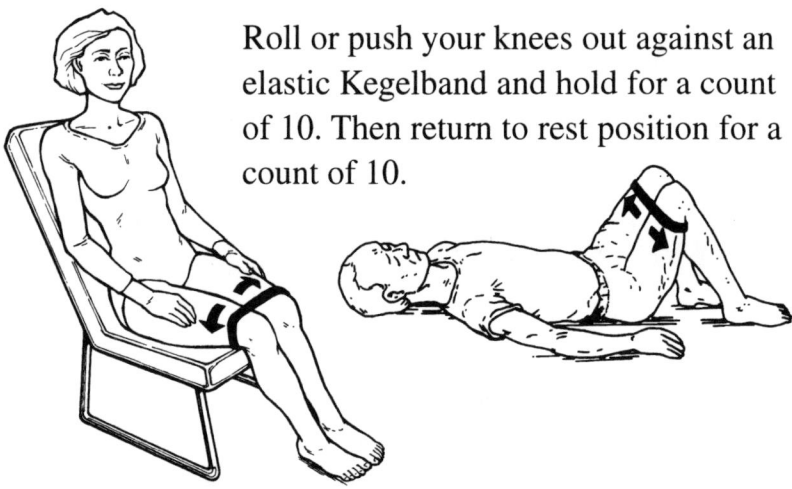

Roll or push your knees out against an elastic Kegelband and hold for a count of 10. Then return to rest position for a count of 10.

Roll your knees in on a Kegelball and hold for a count of 10. Then release pressure to rest for a count of 10.

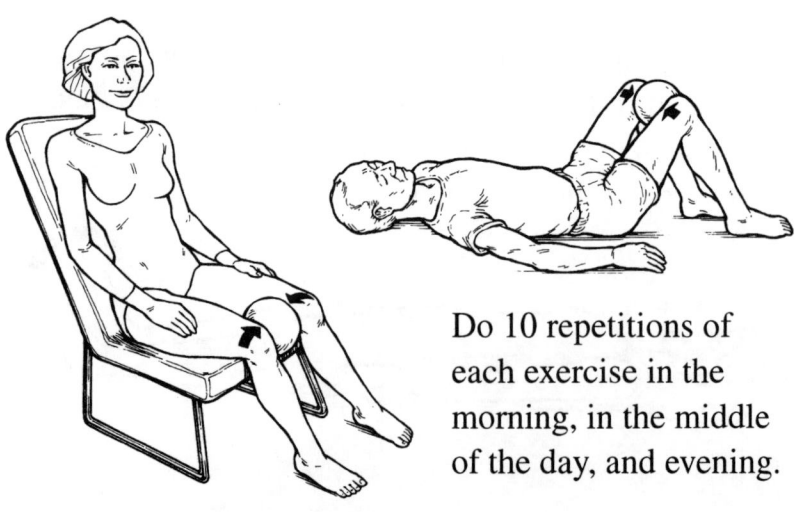

Do 10 repetitions of each exercise in the morning, in the middle of the day, and evening.

BEYOND KEGELS – STANDING PLÍE

Once the first exercise becomes easy, and if you can stand up, add one more exercise.

Stand with your back against a wall and your toes pointing out like a duck. Hold on to a chair for support if needed.

Slowly bend your knees 1-2 inches, then straighten them to the original position. Continue this exercise for 5-10 repetitions a day.

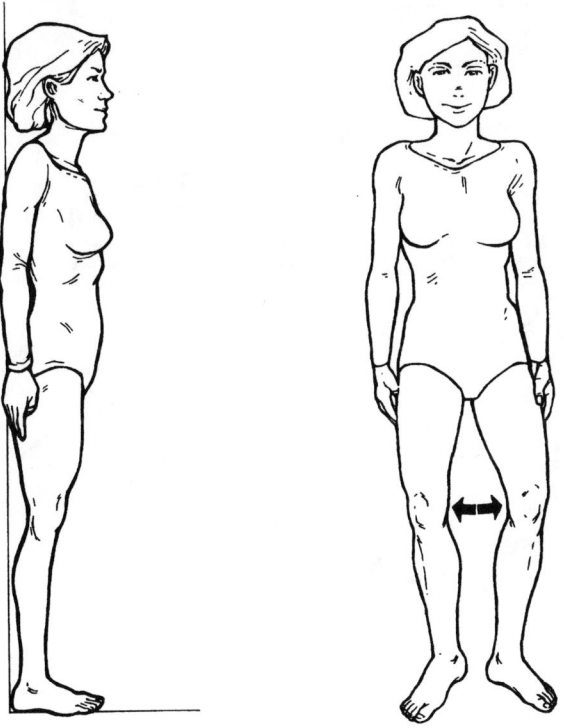

RELAXED AWARENESS OF THE PELVIC MUSCLES

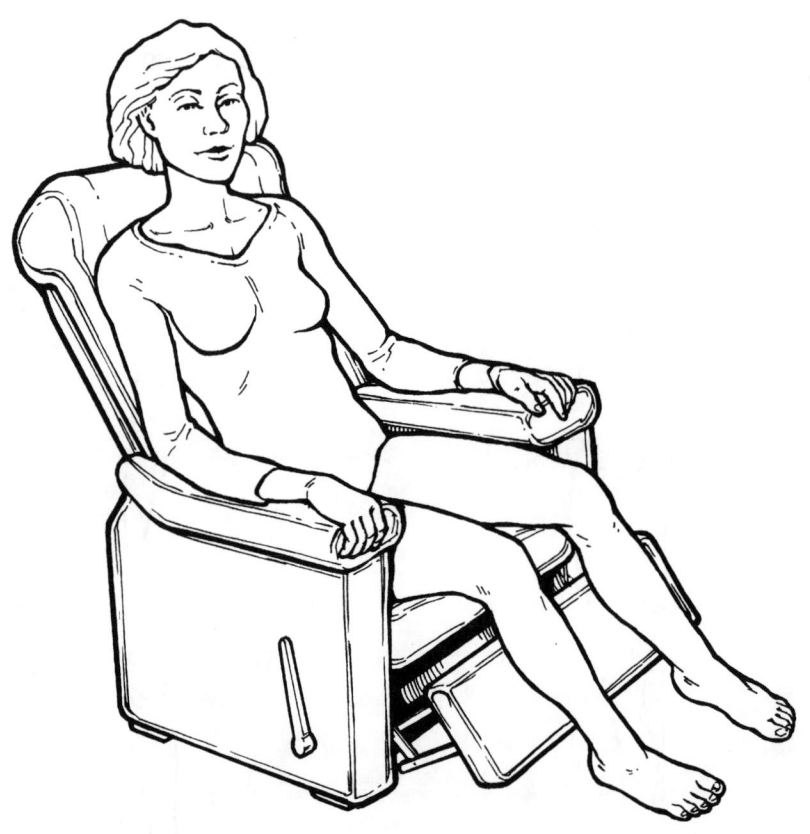

Figure 5-1

BEYOND KEGELS – ACTIVE RESISTIVE EXERCISES
Relaxed Awareness of the Pelvic Muscles

In a comfortable and supported position, either reclining on a bed, in a recliner, or semisitting or sitting in a chair, concentrate on the feel of the support given by the chair or bed from your head down to your feet. Feel that support and relax into that support, release tension into the support through your head and neck, shoulders and back, arms and hands; let your hips and legs sink into the support, let your ankles and feet relax and release into the bed or the chair.

Next, notice your breathing. Notice the natural rhythm of your breathing. Inhale.....Exhale...... Think, "Quiet shoulders, quiet chest." Let your stomach rise with your inhale, fall with your exhale. Now, notice your stomach muscles and your buttocks muscles. Let them be relaxed and totally released as you do these steps. Connect your mind now to the hammock of muscle that forms the base of the pelvis, the hammock of muscle running from the symphysis pubis in the front to the tail bone or coccyx in the back. Maintaining your breathing rhythm, gently tighten this hammock of muscle, gently lift up and in to tighten for a count of 3-5, then release, gently and easily. Try again, tighten and release, maintaining your breathing, keeping your stomach and buttocks relaxed. Do 3 or 4 of these gentle contractions, keeping your mind connected to the hammock of muscle and the support of the chair or bed.

ASSISTED PELVIC MUSCLE TIGHTENING

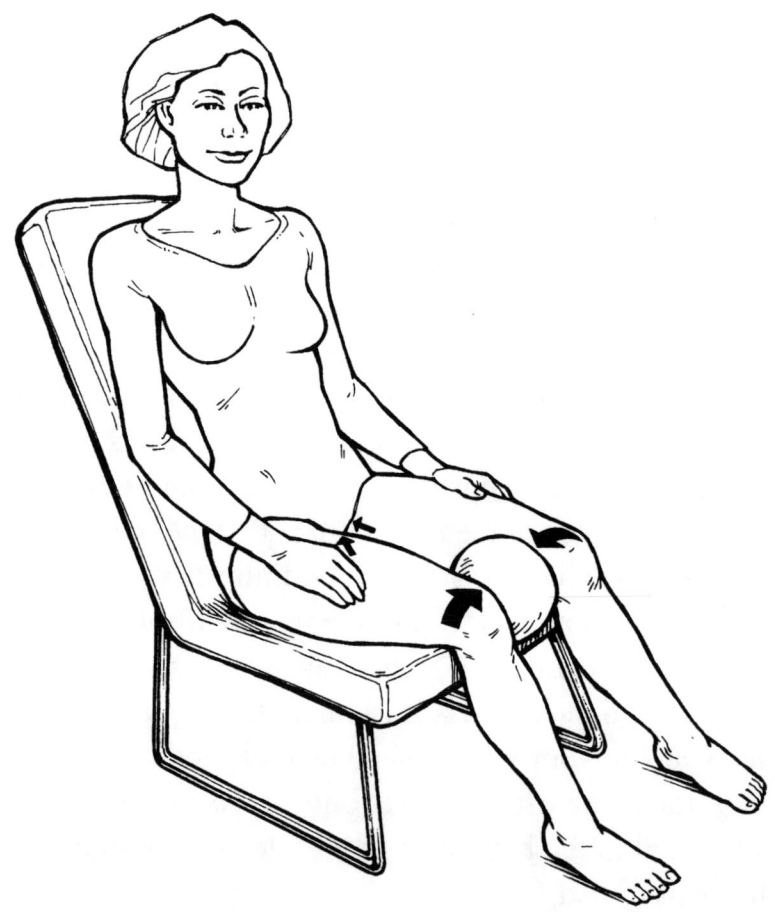

Figure 5-2

Assisted Pelvic Muscle Tightening – Using Adductor/Inner Thigh Muscles

This exercise assists the pelvic diaphragm/levator ani muscles by using the adductor muscles. For this exercise you will be using a Beyond Kegelball. Place the ball between your legs just above the knees. Now roll your knees in against the ball while lifting your pelvic muscles up and in, tightening around the anal and urethral opening, and tightening around the vaginal opening if you are a female. Hold for a count of 10. Now relax and release your knees, the pelvic muscles, your hips and buttocks, your back, neck, and head for a count of 10. Remember as you do this exercise to maintain your breathing rhythm and tighten just the muscles of your inner thighs and the hammock of pelvic muscles. The muscles of your abdomen and buttocks should remain relaxed and loose.

Repeat this exercise 2-3 times a day for 3-5 minutes. If the muscles tire, do them for less time. Continue until this exercise is easy to do. This usually will take 5-7 days.

ASSISTED PELVIC MUSCLE TIGHTENING

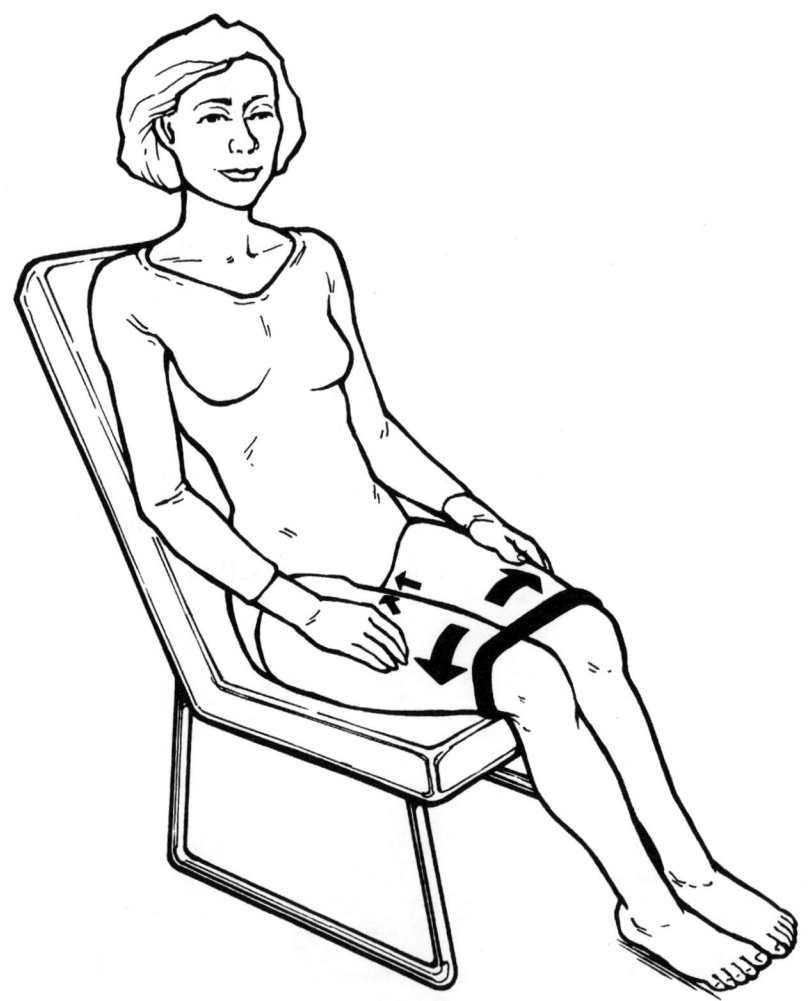

Figure 5-3

**Assisted Pelvic Muscle Tightening –
Using Obturator Internus Muscles/Hip Rotators**

This level of exercise assists the pelvic diaphragm/levator ani muscles by using the obturator internus muscle. In the exercise a Beyond Kegelband, 1-2" wide is secured around your legs just above the knees while the knees are touching. Once secure, roll your knees out against the elastic band while lifting the pelvic muscles up and in, tightening the anal and urethral areas, and vaginal area if appropriate. Count to 10 slowly. Then relax the muscles completely, release your knees, and release your pelvic muscles for a count of 10. Maintaining your breathing rhythm, try this exercise again. Remember that rolling your knees out while using the small hip rotator muscles (the obturator internus) assists the pelvic diaphragm/levator ani muscles in support and stabilization of the bladder, urethra, and bowel.

Repeat this exercise 2-3 times a day for 3-5 minutes. When it is easy to do, progress to the next exercise in this level.

Assisted Pelvic Muscle Tightening – Alternating Inner and Outer Thigh Muscles

Option One

Adductor and obturator muscle assist-exercises can be combined into one. Begin this exercise when the other two assisted exercises are easy to do.

Roll your knees in against the Beyond Kegelball while pulling up and in with the pelvic muscles, holding for a count of 10. Then release and relax for a count of 10.

Now, roll your knees out against the Beyond Kegelband while pulling up and in with the pelvic muscles, and hold for a count of 10. Then relax and release for a count of 10.

Repeat this sequence 2-3 times a day for 3-5 minutes.

Option Two

In any position, hips in neutral position of rotation.
- Roll your legs out as you inhale.
- Let your pelvic muscles relax.
- Let your abdomen rise and your low back arch gently.
- Roll your legs in as you exhale.
- Lift your pelvic muscles up and in, letting your abdomen fall.

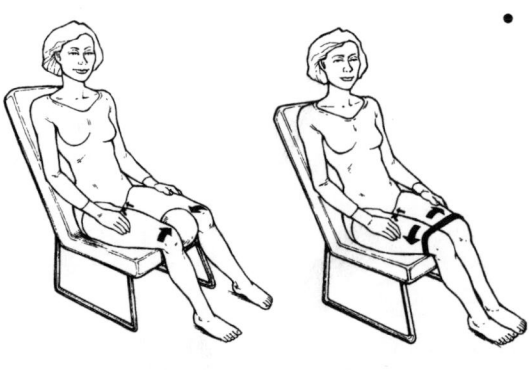

- The abdominals tighten from symphysis pubis to the bellybutton and the low back flattens gently.

Quick Contract and Release of the Pelvic Muscles

The exercise in this level improves the strength and function of the fast acting fibers, primarily of the urogenital diaphragm and external sphincter muscles. These fibers are important for prevention of leaking during coughing, sneezing, lifting, and pulling because these fibers act with speed and intensity to maintain urinary control.

To perform this exercise, focus on your breathing rhythm. Now, maintain that breathing rhythm while you contract the pelvic muscles quickly and forcefully. Tighten at the rectal and urethral openings (vaginal opening if appropriate) simultaneously, and then quickly release. Think or say, "Tighten.....and release." It is as important to release completely and quickly as it is to tighten forcefully. It is also important that the pelvic muscles do the work while the gluteals, abdominals, adductors, and obturator internus muscles remain relaxed.

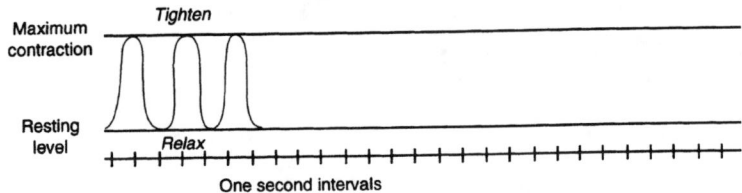

Pelvic Muscle Contraction
Figure 5-4

Perform 5-10 repetitions of this exercise at the beginning and end of each exercise session.

INDEPENDENT PELVIC MUSCLE EXERCISES

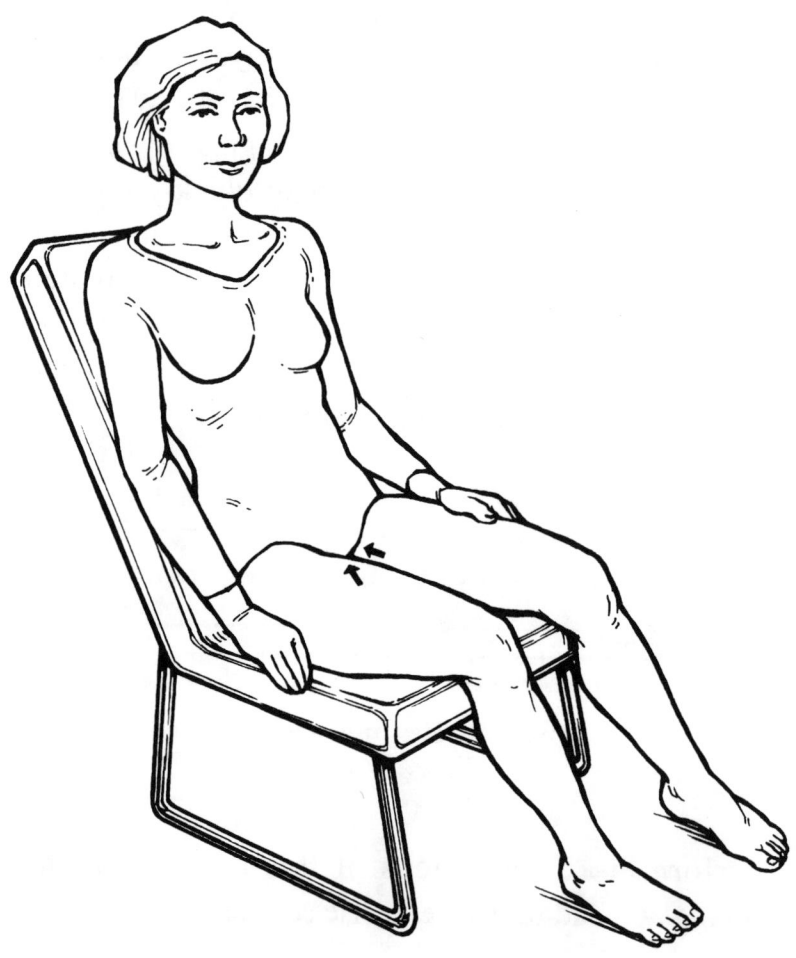

Figure 5-5

Independent Pelvic Muscle Tightening

Tighten (contract) the pelvic muscles, lifting up and in, without tightening any other muscles. Maintain slow, low breathing as you do this. To begin with, pull up and in with the pelvic muscles and hold for a count of 5. Then relax for a count of 10. Notice that you hold this exercise for a count of 5 initially because the pelvic muscles get tired faster when contracting alone. At first they fatigue more. As they become stronger, you can hold for a count of 10 and relax for a count of 10.

Repeat this exercise 4-5 times. Gradually increase the repetitions to 10 as the pelvic muscles become stronger. First, increase the number of seconds you hold the contraction. When you can hold the contractions for 10 seconds, then begin to increase the number of repetitions.

STANDING PLÍE EXERCISE

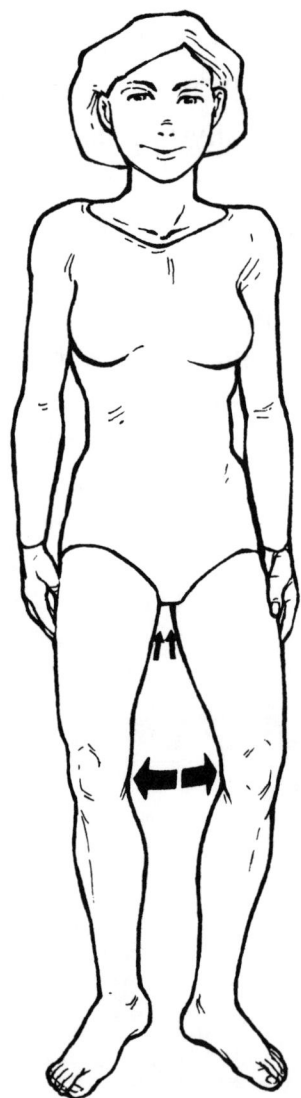

Figure 5-6

Standing Plíe Exercise

Since much of our lives are spent standing, it is important that the pelvic diaphragm/levator ani and obturator internus muscles have adequate strength and endurance to prevent leaking. Performing a small range standing plíe activates the obturator internus-arcuate tendon-levator ani muscles synergistically. In addition, the breathing diaphragm and abdominal muscle action coordinates with the pelvic muscle action to complete the optimal endopelvic support for continence.

Stand with your feet hip width apart with your toes pointing outward. Keep breathing throughout the exercise. Now, for a count of 5, bend the knees 1-2" while tightening the pelvic muscles. Then return to the upright position for a count of 5, keeping the pelvic muscles contracted gently. Relax everything for a count of 10. The knee-bend position with the feet pointed outward brings in the action of the obturator internus-arcuate tendon-pelvic diaphragm/levator ani muscle force field.

Repeat this exercise 3-4 times initially. Gradually increase to 10 repetitions during an exercise session. This is also a good exercise to do while standing in line at the grocery store or movie theater.

ISOLATED PELVIC MUSCLE CONTRACTION IN STANDING

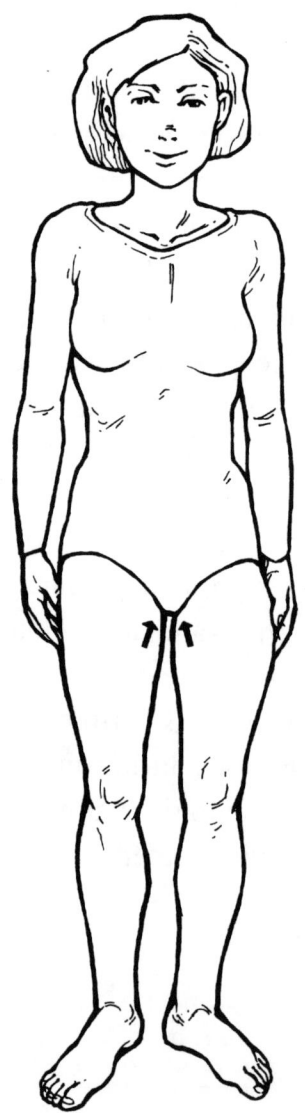

Figure 5-7

Isolated Pelvic Muscle Contraction in Standing

Tighten the pelvic muscles in isolation from all other muscles while in the standing position. Pull up and in while breathing and slowly count to 5, then release and relax muscles for a count of 10. Gradually progress to holding for a count of 10.

Repeat this exercise 3-5 times initially, building up to 10 repetitions over several weeks.

PHYSIOLOGICAL QUIETING

Individuals experiencing incontinence often experience anxiety and fear from their lack of control of bladder and bowel functions. Often when the bladder is overly active the underlying cause is increased activity of the nervous system that is directing bladder function.

The autonomic nervous system directs the bladder in its function and stimulates the symptoms of fear and anxiety (heart racing, fast, shallow breathing, sweaty palms). Often there is an imbalance between sympathetic and parasympathetic portions of the autonomic nervous system. The result can be leaking of urine and poor control of bowel function. If the autonomic nervous system is overactive or on high idle, the bladder sends frequent messages to the brain that it needs to empty and small or large amounts of urine may escape. It is imperative when treating incontinence to use management techniques that quiet the high idle or high resting level of the nervous system innervating the bladder. These techniques are termed Physiological Quieting (PQ). PQ includes the components of diaphragmatic breathing, hand warming, and body/mind quieting.

Diaphragmatic breathing is essential for all individuals and is particularly important for the elderly. As an individual ages, the lungs "forget to exhale" and accumulate carbon dioxide and other waste products deep in the lobes. The exhale phase becomes shallower and shallower. This prevents adequate oxygenated air from being inhaled. When teaching the elderly diaphragmatic breathing, instruct the exhale to be through pursed lips and slightly longer than the inhale. Diaphragmatic breathing quiets the sympathetic fight or flight response. The rhythmic movement of the diaphragm assists in pumping blood and lymph through the abdomen. Diaphragmatic breathing mobilizes the lumbar spine and the visceral organs.

In addition to quieting the body, PQ has the effect of warming the body which can normalize bladder/bowel function. Many older individuals complain that they are cold much of the time. To a large extent the autonomic nervous system determines body warmth by opening or closing blood vessels. Since the autonomic nervous system controls the bladder, bowel, and the blood vessels, when an individual learns to open blood vessels to increase blood flow and keep warm, it also quiets the bladder and bowel, normalizing their function (Fig. 5-11).

Figure 5-11

Relationship of Physiological Quieting–Hand Warming to the AUTONOMIC NERVOUS SYSTEM (ANS), and to the STRIATED AND SMOOTH MUSCLES.

STRIATED MUSCLE

Cognitive Thoughts of Warm Hands ⟶ ANS-Sympathetic-Inhibition

ANS-Sympathetic Inhibition ⟶ Blood Vessel Dilation

Blood Vessel Dilation ⟶ Increased Circulation to Muscles

Increased Circulation to Muscles ⟶ Increased Peripheral Body Temperature
Improved O_2 and Nutrition Delivery
Improved Waste Product Excretion

Cognitive Thoughts of Warm Hands ⟶ ANS-Sympathetic/Parasympathetic Balance

ANS-Sympathetic/Parasympathetic Balance ⟶ Normal Gamma Bias

Normal Gamma Bias ⟶ Normal Striated Muscle Resting Tone

SMOOTH MUSCLE
Cognitive Thoughts of
    Warm Hands ⟶ ANS-Sympathetic/
                                            Parasympathetic
                                            Balance

    ANS-Balance ⟶ Smooth Muscle Quieting
                                   (Bowel, Bladder, Stomach)
                                   Decreased Urge

Diaphragmatic Breathing

The diaphragm is a large sheetlike muscle that rests in a dome shape in the chest cavity from the nipple area to the bottom of the rib cage and the lumbar spine (Fig. 5-12). As you inhale the dome flattens and pulls down to the bottom of the rib cage. During exhale the diaphragm moves back to the dome shape (Fig. 5-13). When breathing correctly, the shoulder and chest areas should remain still and quiet, the jaw is relaxed, and the teeth are separated. The body of the tongue is down and relaxed while the tip touches behind the top front teeth.

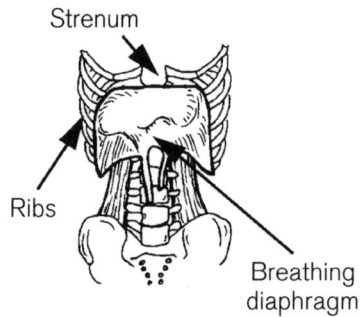

Figure 5-12

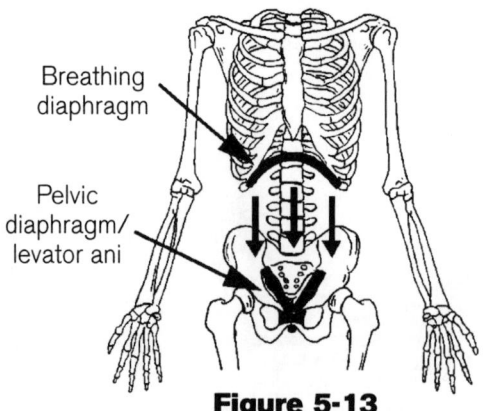

Figure 5-13

To Practice

"Inhale, let your abdomen rise and your low back arch gently. Exhale, let your abdomen fall and your low back flatten. Quiet shoulders, quiet chest."

Inhale through the nose, exhale through the mouth with pursed lips. Exhale for 1 or 2 more counts than inhale.

Practice diaphragmatic breathing initially in a reclined position, then in sitting, and finally a standing position. Practice 4-5 diaphragmatic breaths every hour during the day.

Advanced Diaphragmatic Breathing Technique

In supine focus on your own natural breathing rhythm.

As you inhale
- let your abdomen rise,
- low back gently arch, and
- legs roll out 1-2 inches.

As you exhale
- let your abdomen fall,
- low back gently flatten as the
- lower abdominal muscles gently tighten from symphysis pubis to bellybutton, and
- legs roll in.

After this becomes easy and effortless, you may add the arms by rolling arms out on inhale and rolling them in on exhale.

Hand Warming

Hand warming is a technique to increase blood volume to body parts and quiet the sympathetic portion of the autonomic nervous system. Mental imaging and frequently repeated thoughts transfer to nerve activity that balances the sympathetic (fight or flight) nervous system activity with the parasympathetic resulting in dilation of blood vessels. This autonomic nervous system balance in turn inhibits bladder contractions.

To accomplish this:
1. Focus your attention to your hands and say to yourself, "My hands are warmer and warmer, warmth is flowing into my hands, warmer and warmer."
2. "Think of the warmest color and surround your hands and wrists with that color. Let that color flow into your hands, deep into the fingers, palms, wrists while they get warmer and warmer."
3. "Visualize the warmest place your hands can be: holding a warm cup of hot chocolate, holding your hands over a camp fire or radiator, or slipping your hands and feet in the hot sand of a beach on a summer day."

To accomplish a resetting of the autonomic nervous system, i.e. to slow the high idle, it is necessary to frequently practice the techniques to quiet the sympathetic system for short periods. The instructions are: "Practice hourly for 30-60 seconds" wherever you are. No one will know you are doing it. Put colored dots up around your work and home or wear a watch that buzzes every hour to remind you. Set a kitchen timer or program your computer to remind you.

Then hourly do:
- 7-8 slow, low diaphragmatic breaths.
- 7-8 repetitions of hand warming messages.
- Release jaw, quiet shoulders, quiet chest, relax tongue.

Body/Mind Quieting

Excessive bladder (detrusor) muscle resting tone and increased activity level of bladder and bowel contractions can be decreased through Physiological Quieting of the body and mind, in addition to hand warming techniques previously discussed.

Find a quiet, warm room with a chair or bed that provides complete support from your head to your feet. Use pillows for support of your neck, low back, arms, and knees when needed for comfort.

Then:
1. Focus on your breathing, feel the pattern of breathing, let your abdomen rise with inhale, fall with exhale.
2. Feel the support of the bed or chair and release into that support from the top of your head to the tips of your toes.
3. Focus on your face and neck. Notice where there is any tension or tightness, where there is quiet, calmness in each part of your face and neck. Then,

say to yourself 3-4 times, "My face and neck muscles are quiet and calm, my face and neck muscles are calmer and calmer."
4. Proceed from head to toe in the same manner, focusing on each body part as you did the face and neck.
5. Focus again on diaphragmatic breathing.

One or two 20 minute body/mind quieting sessions a day are recommended. Use the audio tape *Physiological Quieting*.

Integrating Physiological Quieting throughout the day is an essential part of self care for treating incontinence.

CHAPTER 6

BIOFEEDBACK: HOW CAN IT HELP WITH EXERCISES FOR INCONTINENCE?

Take the guesswork out of doing a movement that can't be seen.

Biofeedback measures and displays information occurring within the body, information about muscle activity (electrical activity of muscles), breathing patterns, and hand temperature. This is information a person normally does not perceive, information at an unconscious level. Biofeedback enables an individual to become aware of these processes at a conscious level.

Biofeedback is like a mirror: it shows the individual what the muscles are doing inside the body as they contract and relax. There are many muscles in this region that may be tightened when attempting to tighten the pelvic and urogenital diaphragm muscles. Biofeedback allows an individual to separate one muscle group from the others. Just like the visual image in the mirror, biofeedback brings the image of muscle action to a screen so changes can be made quickly and accurately. If a woman wants to part her hair on the other side or put lipstick on her lips she uses the mirror to tell her first that it needs to be done and second that the changes she made are what she wants and where she wants them. Biofeedback tells the individual what the pelvic muscles are doing in isolation from other muscles, and it shows changes in the action of the muscles immediately and accurately as the individual tightens or relaxes them.

Biofeedback for incontinence is a training method that gives quick, accurate information to the individual about pelvic muscle tightness and muscle relaxation via a computer monitor, a repetitive sound, or a blinking light display. This immediate information improves learning new skills, such as tightening and relaxing pelvic muscles, because it helps the individual make immediate adjustments in the muscle activity.

Biofeedback for incontinence can provide information about the pelvic and urogenital diaphragm muscle groups. Pelvic muscle activity can be monitored directly through sensors recording the electrical activity at the nerve-muscle connection. This is called electromyography (EMG). Surface sensors are applied to the skin surface over the muscle group. When an internal vaginal or anal sensor is used it is inserted like a tampon or suppository in the vagina or anus to pick up pelvic muscle activity closer to the muscle surface. Surface sensors can also monitor abdominal, gluteal, adductor, and breathing diaphragm muscles.

Sensors pick up even slight contractions of the pelvic and urogenital diaphragm muscles when the individual tries to tighten them, and the intensity and pattern of the contraction is visible immediately on the biofeedback display. When a stronger contraction of the same muscles is attempted the observable difference between the two pictures provides reinforcement for improved function of the pelvic muscles. As Martha said during her first biofeedback session, "Oh, so this is how it is supposed to feel when I do the exercise! I thought I was doing it right before, but I wasn't using the right muscles." The feel of the exercise is paired with the objective picture on the screen so changes are made more quickly. The guesswork is taken out of doing a movement that cannot be seen. Problems with stress and urge incontinence and fecal incontinence can be helped with this type of biofeedback. Nonrelaxing puborectalis syndrome can also be treated effectively with biofeedback.

The bladder (detrusor) muscle is not under our voluntary control, but an individual can learn to quiet the bladder's contractions through biofeedback that indirectly monitors the autonomic or "automatic" nervous system that controls the bladder. Although it is not possible to directly control the bladder, a general quieting of the autonomic nervous system will quiet the bladder. Because this nervous system also controls breathing rate and circulation, if an individual learns to slow the breathing rate or warm the hands by increasing the blood flow to the hands, there is a crossover effect to the bladder. The bladder quiets so the frequent urge to urinate passes as the individual's breathing slows and hands warm. Sensors that pick up hand temperature tell the individual if the circulation is improving by showing the rising temperature on a monitor (for example from 86.5°F. to 88.7°F.). Sensors that measure movement of the diaphragm tell the individual how many breaths per minute occur, and how effectively the diaphragm muscle activity increases and decreases on the monitor. Problems with urge incontinence and an unstable bladder can be helped using this type of biofeedback.

Biofeedback can be used at home as well as in the clinic. Small home units are available that have their own light bars or small screens. The sensors are easy to use for the once-or-twice a day practice sessions. Some home units can "download" into the clinic computer; that is, they store information about practice session frequency and results, which then is transferred to the clinic computer.

Biofeedback can be used successfully if an individual is able to process information through sight or sound and make modifications based on that input. It is necessary, however, that the individual be motivated and wants to learn the exercise prescribed. There are no side effects and biofeedback can be noninvasive.

Biofeedback in conjunction with therapeutic exercise has been shown to be more effective and faster in diminishing incontinence than exercise alone. Biofeedback gives more accurate, fast information to the brain which improves the learning curve, increases muscle strength more quickly, and reintegrates reflex arcs more completely.

CHAPTER 7

LIFE STYLE CHANGES FOR CONTINENCE

An elderly individual with leaking problems changes his/her behavior to accommodate the leaking. Changes may occur in:
1. Clothing worn.
2. Location and supplies used for sleep.
3. Activities inside and outside the home.
4. Food and drink consumed.
5. Frequency of toileting.
6. Friendships that are maintained.
7. Intimate relationships that are maintained.
8. Recreational or exercise activities engaged in.
9. Changes in self-concept and self-acceptance.

CLOTHING

An individual experiencing incontinence will often wear only dark or black pants or skirts to hide any wetness. Clothing has to be cleaned often, so washable clothing must be purchased. Taking a change of clothes wherever one goes is easier if they are wash-and-wear and lightweight so they can dry quickly and fit in a tote bag. Pants that are easily removed are important so leaking doesn't occur due to the delay caused by removing clothing.

Specialized, protective, reusable underwear are often worn in conjunction with incontinence pads. Other times, disposable briefs with absorbent pads are helpful. Some individuals use toweling, toilet paper, or sanitary pads to absorb leaks in regular underwear (see Chapter 14).

NIGHTTIME

Some individuals have leaking problems at night. Various means of protection are used including an absorbent bed pad, a towel placed on the bed, or specialized underwear and pads. It is important to have appropriate protection so the individual can sleep through the night without the fear of wetting the bed. The frail elderly need to have pad and position changes during the night but voiding frequency may decrease so changing can often be every 3-4 hours instead of every 2 hours.

If leaking at night is prevalent, then some independent elderly report moving from sleeping with a partner to sleeping alone until the problem diminishes. Although difficult, it is important to communicate with a partner about feelings and facts as well as listening to his/her needs before the change is made.

At times, elderly individuals get up to toilet more than 2 times per night. Sleep is severely disrupted and stress increases. Physiological Quieting at bedtime and/or when the individual awakens in the night helps alleviate this problem. When an individual wakes up with the urge to urinate using the urge protocol strategies before getting up, a bedside commode or urinal may be appropriate. Eliminating fluid intake after six in the evening may also extend the sleep time.

FOOD AND DRINK

One of the most common comments heard when an elderly individual has a leaking problem is, "I quit drinking much so I won't leak." Decreasing liquid intake decreases bladder size because the bladder stretches or shrinks depending on how much fluid is in it on a regular basis. As the bladder shrinks from the decreased amount of fluid being consumed, the brain is told that the bladder is "full" more frequently and the brain tells the bladder to empty the urine more frequently. The result can be toileting routines that are every 30-60 minutes instead of the normal routine of every 2-4 hours. Less fluid also concentrates the urine which results in irritation to the bladder wall. This often sets off bladder contractions. Instead of the common misconception that less fluid decreases leaking, the reality is that less fluid increases frequency of urination and bladder irritability, which often leads to more leaking. Therefore, drinking adequate fluid, 6-8 glasses per day, is recommended.

Alcoholic beverages are not recommended because they alter the nervous system's ability to control the bladder and bowel function and can be a bladder irritant. Alcohol also functions as a diuretic. It is therefore important for individuals experiencing incontinence to eliminate alcoholic beverages from their diet.

Caffeine is also a highly irritating substance to the nervous system that controls the bladder and bowel. The residue it leaves in urine acts as a bladder irritant. Eliminating caffeine, including coffee, sodas, teas, and chocolate, can decrease or eliminate incontinence. Citrus fruits can also be an irritant to the bladder.

Some elderly individuals are negatively affected by highly spiced foods or citrus fruits, still others are sensitive to milk or wheat products. An elimination diet of 7-10 days can determine if the incontinence symptoms are related to a specific food product.

Some elderly individuals will use food as an emotional support when there is embarrassment and loss of control stemming from incontinence. Increased weight of even five pounds can have a significant impact on increasing incontinence. Inadequate food intake with the resulting weight loss leads to nutritional deficiencies that affect bladder and bowel function as well.

TOILETING FREQUENCY

Increased toileting frequency is a common adaptation to leaking. Toileting before going out of the house is another adaptation to incontinence. The thought is if one toilets more often then there won't be leaking. Frequent toileting leads to decreased bladder size and an even more frequent need to urinate. Toileting before going anywhere becomes a conditioned response so it becomes impossible to go anywhere without toileting. It is important to space toiletings approximately 2-4 hours apart. If there is an urge to urinate before the 2-hour interval, following an urge protocol will assist in extending the time between toileting (see p. 73).

FRIENDSHIPS

Isolation can be a problem when the individual with incontinence is embarrassed by the urine loss and is fearful someone will notice an offensive odor, a wet spot on his/her clothes, the bulge of pads used, or the frequency with which she/he uses the toilet. The ultimate fear is a major accident when with friends or in public. It is important not to let these fears interfere with social activity. Outings with friends and family are essential to a happy, healthy life. The elderly can feel secure if they plan ahead and wear comfortable clothing, bring a change of clothing, wear pads or protective undergarments. It is important for the elderly to do whatever is necessary to be with friends and family.

It is important to tell friends about a leaking problem in a brief but informative way. "My bladder needs special attention so I need to use the bathroom frequently," is what Madeline told her friend when they went shopping. Speaking up the first time is often the hardest but it is important to maintain friendships since isolation leads to depression in even the healthiest person. Linda shared how she viewed her problem: "Incontinence is no different than poor eyesight. I use pads and do exercises for my leaking problem just like I wear glasses to improve my eyesight. Then I get on with my life, love, and happiness."

INTIMATE RELATIONSHIPS

Intimate relationships are an important consideration when dealing with incontinence. The partner in an established relationship needs to be informed about the problem and possible solutions in order to maintain physical and emotional closeness. Sharing feelings, both positive and negative, helps both partners continue the relationship. The questions, "How do you feel about this leaking?" "What are the aspects you are comfortable with?" "What parts make you feel uncomfortable?" are good to pose to a partner. It is important to follow those questions with active listening and answering questions in a straight forward manner.

Expanding the definition of intimacy can be helpful in any relationship. Sometimes leaking occurs during intercourse. Using a plastic mattress pad or having intercourse in the hot tub or shower are options. Changing positions from the missionary position to sidelying or all fours with rear entry may put less pressure on the bladder.

Intimacy also includes physical hugging, caresses, and kissing; it can be verbal expressions of caring, it can be music. Intimacy can be movement in the form of dance, it can be fragrances in the environment, it can be the written word (25 reasons I love you), or a daily special note at the breakfast table. Intimacy can take many forms when we open our minds and hearts to love and it should never be disrupted by a little leaking.

RECREATIONAL ACTIVITIES

Maintaining an active and enjoyable life style is an important aspect in treating incontinence. Physical exercise is vital to emotional and physical health. Physical exercise increases the endorphins–chemicals that elevate mood and are often called the "good humor hormones." Physical activity increases metabolism to help maintain weight control. Physical activity tones and strengthens muscles throughout the body.

Too often, physical exercise is eliminated in an attempt not to leak. As 65-year-old Judy commented, "When I walk any distance I leak, so I quit walking except around the house." Rather than quitting a favorite activity, it is important to make adaptations in order to continue the activity without embarrassment. Use of a superabsorbent pad can enable physical activity. Taking breaks allows time for toileting when needed. Bringing extra clothing in case an accident occurs is also important. Incontinence can also be the impetus to try new activities.

SELF-CONCEPT AND SELF-ESTEEM

Feelings of shame and embarrassment about leaking often become generalized to the whole person, negatively affecting self-esteem. Common symptoms of depression include sadness, lack of energy, change in eating habits, and sleep disruption. Identifying with infantile or aging behavior rather than healthy, active adult behavior may be experienced. Confidence can turn to feelings of vulnerability, frustration, and anger. Examples of negative self-talk include, "I smell repulsive," "I can't go anywhere if the toilet isn't close by," "I act like a baby and treat myself like one," "If I were a stronger person, I could control this leaking," "My body is going downhill, losing control, and soon I'll be ready for the graveyard."

Active coping strategies are essential to positive self-esteem and self-concept. Encourage the elderly individual to:

1. Admit and identify the leaking problem.
2. Assertively gather information about the specific

problem. Consult books, physicians, support groups, and the internet.
3. Consider all possible solutions before making an educated decision about the route to take.
4. Develop and practice positive self-statements, such as, "I can make adaptations and go wherever I want," "I am an active, energetic adult who can solve a leaking problem," "I am a special person who deserves the best."
5. Practice self-reliance while asking for assistance when needed to change life style habits that will facilitate being independent and continent.

GETTING STARTED AND KEEPING TRACK OF CHANGES

To begin life style changes, the individual is encouraged to pick two or three of the ideas just discussed and implement them. For instance:

Eliminate all caffeine and alcohol, including colas, coffee, and chocolate.

Drink six to eight glasses of fluid a day to maintain the size of the bladder and also to dilute the concentration of urine.

Do some fun and moderate aerobic activity every day. Twenty minutes of walking, swimming or stationary biking daily will help to strengthen the pelvic muscles and maintain overall good health.

To see progress, keep a daily journal. Record the glasses of fluid consumed, the caffeine consumed, the activity participated in, and the amount of time spent on the activity.

LIFE STYLE CHANGES FOR CONTINENCE
Adequate Fluid
- Six to eight glasses noncaffeinated fluid daily interspersed throughout the day.
- Water (add lemon/lime slices), diluted fruit juice, no soda/pop.

Eliminate Caffeine and Alcohol
- No coffee, tea, chocolate (eliminate gradually).
- It is a bladder and nervous system irritant.

Use Positive Self Statements
- I am an active, energetic adult who can solve a leaking problem.

Eliminate Tight Clothing
- It can irritate the bladder.
- It is hard to get off to toilet.

Moderate Aerobic Activity
- 20-30 minutes daily, not measured in speed or endurance.
- Walking, biking, swimming, etc.
- Coordinates pelvic muscles with functional activity.
- Improves neuromuscular coordination.
- Improves total body/mind well-being.

Pacing Work/Rest Cycles
- Rest periods during the day so pelvic muscles are gravity free.

- Physiological Quieting for autonomic nervous system balance.
- Minimum 2-3 rest periods/day.
- Use Physiological Quieting during rest.

Fun/Laughter
- 1-3 bouts daily.
- Read the funnies, tell a joke, watch a funny video.

WHAT TO DO WHEN YOU HAVE THE URGE?

When the urge to urinate hits, when the key is in the door and you don't think you can make it fast enough to the bathroom, what do you do?

- Stand quietly with relaxed posture.
- Consciously relax the abdominal muscles.
- Breathe slow and low, 3-4 breaths
- Visualize a quiet and peaceful place.
- Say to yourself: "My bladder is calm, my abdomen is relaxed."
- Tighten the pelvic muscles 4-5 times in quick contractions or roll legs in and out 4-5 times.
- Continue to the bathroom after the urge has quieted if it has been 2-3 hours since the last toileting.

CHAPTER 8

WHAT MEDICATIONS CAN HELP?

Medications have been shown to be beneficial in treating urinary incontinence. In conjunction with exercise and behavioral strategies, they are recommended as an appropriate treatment for incontinence in the Clinical Practice Guideline published by the Department of Health and Human Services, 1996.

Short term medication trials benefit some patients with urge incontinence, but the side effects can be significant and research indicates that few individuals become symptom-free.

Medication use may improve symptoms in approximately half of the individuals with stress or mixed incontinence, but again few become symptom-free. Medications used for stress incontinence have fewer side effects than those used for urge incontinence.

Medications used for overflow incontinence exhibit significant side effects, and improvement in symptoms varies.

Medication use should be based on individual patient needs, i.e., contraindications, cost, and drug interactions. Initial dosages in most medications used for incontinence should be low and increased slowly.

Pharmacologic treatment for urinary incontinence is an important component of treatment but best results often occur when used in combination with exercise, behavioral, and sometimes surgical strategies.

Medications Used to Relieve Incontinence
Urge Incontinence
    Anticholinergic Agents
        oxybutynin (Ditropan) (Ditropan XL)
        dicyclomine hydrochloride (Bentyl)
        propantheline (Pro-Banthine)
        hyoscyamine (Levsin)
        tolterodine tartrate (Detrol)
    Estrogen Replacement Therapy (ERT)
    Tricyclic Antidepressant Agents
        imipramine (Tofranil)
        doxepin (Sinequan)
        desipramine (Norpramin)
        nortriptyline (Pamelor)
        amitriptyline (Elavil)

Stress Incontinence
Alpha Adrenergic Agonists
    phenylpropanolamine (PPA)
Estrogen Replacement Therapy (ERT)
Combination Therapy
    tricyclic antidepressant agents
    and antidiuretic hormone

Overflow Incontinence
Alpha Adrenergic Antagonists
    terazosin (Hytrin)
    prazosin (Minipress)
    doxazosin (Cardura)
Cholinergic Agonists
    bethanechol (Urecholine)

Description of Commonly Used Medications
Urge Incontinence
   Anticholinergic Agents
      Function: Decreases bladder contractions, relaxes smooth muscle
      Effect: Decreases urge incontinence leaking, increases bladder capacity, increases time between voiding

Examples:	*Dose*
oxybutynin (Ditropan)	2.5-5 mg
(Ditropan XL)	1-4x/day
propantheline (Pro-Banthine)	7.5-30 mg, 15-60mg
dicyclomine hydrochloride (Bentyl)	20 mg 4x/day
hyoscyamine (Levsin)	0.125-0.25 mg 3-4 x/day
tolterodine tartrate (Detrol)	1-2 mg 2x/day

      Side effects: Dry skin, blurred vision, change in mental state, drowsiness, confusion, nausea, constipation, dry mouth, tachycardia (increased heart rate), weakness, orthostatic hypotension (low blood pressure on arising from reclining)
      Note: Should not be used if narrow angle glaucoma is present.

   Estrogen Replacement Therapy (ERT)

   Tricyclic Antidepressant Agents (TCA)
      Function: Increases CNS serotonin neurotransmitter levels
      Effect: Reduces daytime leaking, reduces nighttime leaking

Examples	*Dose*
imipramine (Tofranil)	10-25 mg 1-4x/day
doxepin (Sinequan)	10-50 mg 3x/day
desipramine (Norpramin)	25 mg 1-3x/day

nortriptyline (Pamelor)   10-25 mg 1-3x/day
amitriptyline (Elavil)   10-25 mg 3-4x/day
Side effects: cardiac alterations, anticholinergic effects, fatigue, xerostomia, dizziness, blurred vision

Stress Incontinence

Alpha Adrenergic Agonists
Function: Affects receptors at bladder neck, internal sphincter, and proximal urethra causing muscle contraction in this area
Effect: Decreases leaking with intra-abdominal pressure, tightens bladder outlet muscle
Examples   *Dose*
phenylpropanolamine   25-50 mg 4x/day
(PPA) (Dexatrim)
psuedoephedrine (Sudafed)   30-60 mg 4x/day
Side Effects: Nausea, xerostomia, insomnia, restlessness, anxiety, headache, hypertension, heart palpitations
Note: Not to be used in people with increased blood pressure/hypertension, severe congestive heart failure, cardiac arrhythmias

Estrogen Replacement Therapy(ERT)
Function: Restore urethral mucosa, increase vascularity, tone and responsiveness of urethral muscle, increase alpha adrenergic receptors of urethra
Effect: Improve internal sphincter function, decrease incontinence with increased intra-abdominal pressure, decreases irritative voiding symptoms, decreases frequency of urination especially at night
Examples   *Dose*
conjugated estrogen   0.623-1.25 mg daily
(Premarin)
Side Effects: Not recommended for women with a history of breast or uterine cancer, blood clots, or liver damage

Combination Therapy–ERT and PPA
> Recommended in stress incontinence in post-menopausal women if single drug therapy has proven inadequate

Tricyclic Antidepressant Agents
> imipramine (Tofranil)   75 mg/day
> (See description under Urge Incontinence medications.)
> (Propranolol and other beta blockers are not recommended at this time due to lack of clinical research.)
> Antidiurectic Hormone
> desmopressin (DDAVP)
> *Effect:* Decreases nocturnal enuresis (nighttime wetting) and nighttime polyuria; at this time used for children only

Overflow Incontinence

Alpha Adrenergic Antagonists
> *Function:* Relaxes internal sphincter muscle
> *Effect:* Increases outlet size causing improved flow of urine, decreased residual urine, decreased leaking due to more complete emptying
>
> | *Examples* | *Dose* |
> |---|---|
> | terazosin (Hytrin) | 1 mg daily |
> | prazosin (Minipress) | 1 mg 2-3x/daily |
> | doxazosin (Cardura) | 1 mg daily |
>
> *Side Effects:* Orthostatic hypotension (which can lead to falls, should be taken at bedtime), tachycardia (increased heart rate)

Cholinergic Agonists
> *Function:* Increases bladder muscle contractions
> *Effect:* Increases force with which bladder muscle pushes urine down and out the urethra, decreases residual urine, decreases leaking because of more complete emptying

Example   *Dose*
bethanechol (Urecholine)   10-50 mg 2-4x/day
Side Effects: flushing, abdominal cramps, diarrhea, nausea and vomiting, sweating, salivation

Medications that Cause Incontinence Symptoms

Many of the same medications used to treat incontinence can also cause incontinence if used inappropriately. Medications used to treat other conditions can have side effects that cause incontinence.

Medication	**Possible Side Effects**
Sedatives/Hypnotics	sedation, immobility, muscle relaxation

CNS Depressants
    diazepan (Valium)
    flurazepam (Dalmane)
    alcohol
	delirium, frequency and urgeency leaking

Diuretics
    furosemide (Lasix)
    bumetanide (Bumex)
    loop diuretics
	polyuria, frequency and urgency leaking

Antipsychotics
    thioridazine (Mellaril)
    haloperidol (Haldol)
	sedation, rigidity, immobility, urge and overflow leaking, anticholinergic actions

Antidepressants
    imiprimine (Tofranil)
    doxepin (Sinequan)
    desipramine (Norpramin)
    amitriptyline (Elavil)
	fatigue, dizziness, bladder relaxation, constipation

Anti-Parkinson Agents
   benztropine (Cogentin)
   trihexyphenidyl (Artane)
	bladder relaxation,
	urge and overflow leaking

Anticholinergic Agents
   antihistamines—
   diphenhydramine
   (Benadryl)
   hydroxyzine
   (Vistaril, Atarax)
	sedation, urine retention,
	weak stream,
	frequency,
	urge and overflow leaking,
	fecal impaction

Alpha Adrenergic Agonist Agents
   phenylpropranolamine
   (Ephedrine)
	sedation, urine retention,
	weak stream, frequency,
	urge and overflow leaking

Alpha Adrenergic Antagonist Agents
   prazosin (Minipress)
   terazosin (Hytrin)
   doxazosin (Cardura)
	urethral relaxation,
	leak with cough/
	sneeze/laugh

Calcium Channel Blocking Agents
   nifedipine
   (Adalat, Procardia)
   diltiazem (Cardizem)
	urine retention,
	fluid retention,
	bladder (detrusor)
	relaxation

Narcotic Analgesic Agents morphine, etc.	urine retention, sedation, delirium, fecal impaction
Antihypertensive Agents	bladder and sphincter relaxation
Caffeine	aggravation or precipitation of leaking

CHAPTER 9

CONFIDENT AND CONTINENT PREVENTION PROGRAM

It is just as important to prevent incontinence from occurring in the aging population as it is to treat it when it occurs. A continence prevention program can have more impact in the elderly than in any other age group since its implications in socialization and independence are significant.

The prevention program involves nutritional, exercise, and Physiological Quieting techniques. Increasing fluid intake to six to eight glasses daily helps to maintain adequate bladder size and keep urine diluted. Eliminating caffeine quiets the autonomic nervous system that innervates the bladder and eliminates bladder irritating chemicals. Vitamin B12 is often depleted in older individuals with urine retention problems. Vitamin B12 depletion can lead to depression so injections and/or supplements are often recommended. An effective bowel program is needed in most older individuals to maintain regular, effective bowel movements. This secondarily helps with normal bladder function since bowel and bladder are innervated by the same nervous system and anatomically are in close proximity to each other (see p. 26 for bowel program). Moderate aerobic exercise (walking is best) improves general well being and stimulates pelvic muscle force field action and normal bowel/colon activity. Beyond Kegels exercises facilitate support and function of the internal organs. Physiological Quieting helps to normalize the autonomic nervous system that controls the bladder and bowel.

CONFIDENT & CONTINENT PREVENTION PROGRAM

- Caffeine Eliminated_____ cups/day
- Non Caffeinated Fluid/Day – 6-8 glasses
- Vitamin B12
- Effective Bowel Program
  Fluid___, Fiber___, Vitamin C____, Magnesium___, Massage___

PHYSIOLOGICAL QUIETING
Hand Warming/Diaphragmatic Breathing
- Focus on warmth in your hands.
- Think to yourself, "My hands are warmer & warmer."
- "Warmth is flowing into my hands, warmer & warmer."
- Inhale as your bellybutton rises.
- Exhale as your bellybutton falls.
- Maintain relaxed jaw, tongue, and shoulders.
- Repeat 5-7 times hourly.

Body/Mind Quieting
- *Physiological Quieting* audiotape at bedtime.

MODERATE AEROBIC ACTIVITY –
- 20-30 minutes/day walking, biking, pool.

BEYOND KEGELS EXERCISES (5-10 repetitions)
Assisted Pelvic Muscle Tightening – Adductors

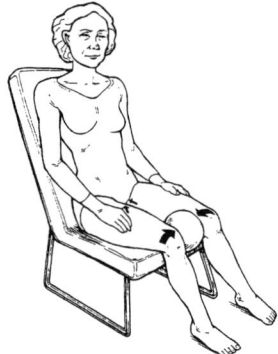

- Roll your knees in on a Kegelball as you lift up and in with pelvic muscles.
- Hold for 10 counts, release for 10 counts.

Assisted Pelvic Muscle Tightening – Obturators

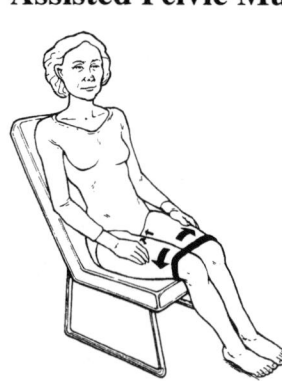

- Roll your legs out against Beyond Kegelband as you lift up and in with pelvic muscles.
- Hold for 10 counts, release for 10 counts.

Standing Plíe

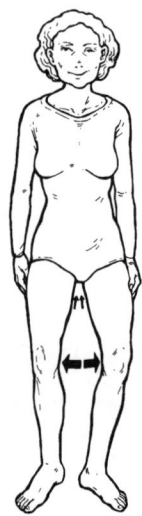

- Stand with feet pointing outward, hip width apart.
- Slowly bend knees 1-2" as you inhale for a count of 5.
- Straighten knees as you exhale for a count of 5.
- Repeat for 10 repetitions.

CHAPTER 10

THE ACTIVE ELDERLY AT HOME AND INDEPENDENT

THE ACTIVE ELDERLY

Over ninety percent of individuals 65 and older live independently in their own residence. Bladder and bowel continence is an important function in maintaining their independence. The active elderly individual often describes problems leaking with increased intra-abdominal pressure when he/she arises from a bed or chair, when walking any distance, when bending down, or when pushing or pulling an object. Leaking is often experienced with laughing, coughing, and sneezing.

The active elderly describe leaking with the sudden feeling of urge caused by the bladder muscle being overactive or irritated. Urge leaking can occur with the key in the door after having been shopping, when turning on the water in the kitchen or bath, when going out into cold air, or when putting hands in the freezer. Sometimes urge leaking occurs at the bathroom door–just inches away from the toilet. Some individuals check often to see if the need to toilet is present. The act of checking may "set off" an urge feeling. Checking if done, should be only at every 2-3 hour intervals.

The active elderly describe an increasing frequency of toileting during the day and night. Factors of nighttime increased frequency of urination or leaking include increased renal blood flow and increased venous return in the supine position, increased diuresis at night in the elderly, and circadian rhythm changes with age. This increased bladder activity means the elderly individual is more wakeful at night and thus sleepy during the daytime. The frequency of toileting may be self initiated to "prevent leaking" or it may occur spontaneously from an urge feeling.

Often elderly turn to "just in case" toileting. However, the "just in case" toileting to prevent leaking is counter productive, leading to smaller and smaller bladder size. When toileting occurs more frequently than every 2-3 hours during the day or 1-2 times per night it interferes with freedom to participate in daily activities and quality and quantity of sleep. As the frequency increases the urine often becomes more concentrated and irritates the bladder leading to more irritation. Relatively easy procedures can increase the time between toileting day and night (see p. 73 Urge Protocol).

Decreasing fluid intake is one of the most common responses of the elderly to any symptoms of leaking, urge, or toileting frequency. This only compounds a natural decrease in water intake with age and can lead to serious dehydration. The nervous system innervation of the GI tract decreases with age making swallowing slower and more difficult, especially swallowing thin liquids like water. The elderly choke or gag on thin liquids more frequently and thus may avoid them. The elderly gradually lose the automatic thirst for water when the body needs it and thus there is not the natural tendency to pick up a glass of water to drink. The aging body tissues tend to hold fluid and diurese or release the fluid from the tissues when the individual reclines or sits for a period of time. Thus, relatively large amounts of urine may occur periodically during the day instead of smaller amounts throughout the day. This combination of factors can lead to dehydration, to more acidic concentrated urine, and/or to constipation. Adequate fluid intake is essential for continence and health in the elderly. It must be a planned event throughout the day.

Medications can cause or contribute to urinary and bowel incontinence symptoms. Diuretics, narcotics, analgesics, antidepressants, antihistamines, and alpha adrenergic agonists and antagonists can impact continence (see p. 79). Discussions with a physician can lead to changes in medication or changes in medication schedule that may help the incontinence symptoms. For example, a diuretic given at half dose two times daily may eliminate incontinence symptoms brought on by a whole dose given once daily.

Constipation or fecal impaction has a significant role in urinary incontinence. Assessing and managing bowel problems often will lead to improved function of both systems (see p. 23). Other transient causes of incontinence are discussed in Chapter 3.

When leaking or the fear of leaking is present the use of appropriate protection is paramount for the individual to continue active daily activities, recreation, and social schedules. Many types of protection are available, from light mini pads appropriate for a few lost drops to super absorbency pads for continuous large leaks. Disposable pads and disposable and reusable undergarments with absorbent pads are available in grocery stores, pharmacies, and through mail order (see Resources p. 165). An important aspect of a continence program is selecting appropriate, comfortable protective pads/undergarments and gradually changing the absorbancy level and type as continence improves. The fear of leaking leads some individuals to wear excess protection when it is not needed.

Life style changes occur with leaking or the fear of leaking in public places and when others are around. Chapter Seven discusses positive approaches to address these limiting factors effectively.

Active men as they age may have urge, retention, and/or incontinence symptoms secondary to conditions such as prostate enlargement or prostatectomy. Chapter Twelve describes conditions and treatment approaches for men.

A self-administered questionnaire can be the initial screening device to determine if incontinence is a problem. A more in-depth history and medical evaluation is done by a health professional when screening indicates problems.

Questions important to answer include:
    1. How would you describe your leaking?

2. How long have you had the leaking problem?
3. When does it occur?
4. How often do you leak urine during the day? During the night?
5. What makes it worse? What makes it better?
6. How have you changed your life because of leaking?
7. Do you have trouble getting to the bathroom on time? What situations?
8. Do you leak if you cough, sneeze, lift, run, or jump?
9. Do you leak when arising from a chair or a bed?
10. How frequently do you toilet during the day? At night?
11. What prompts you to go to the toilet?
12. When toileting is there a strong or weak stream?
13. Does urine stop and start easily and completely?
14. How often do you have a bowel movement?
15. Do you have problems with constipation or diarrhea?
16. What type of protection do you use?
17. How much fluid do you consume daily? What kinds?
18. What is the pattern of your fluid consumption?
19. Have you changed your fluid consumption since leaking started?
20. How much caffeine do you consume daily?
21. Have you had frequent bladder infections?
22. Do you experience pain or irritation with urination?

23. Is there blood in your urine?
24. What, if any, medications are you taking?
25. What surgeries have you had?

The next step is to evaluate a three to seven day bladder/bowel record that includes information on toileting frequency, leaking episodes, fluid intake, and amount of protection used. If bladder retention is a potential problem, 24-hour urine output should also be measured.

DAILY RECORD

The first step is to keep a bladder/bowel record for several days or a week. The bladder/bowel record will provide current information on toileting frequency, leaking episodes, fluid intake, and amount of protection used.

Under each day there are two-hour blocks of time. Record a "TU" each time you urinate in the toilet, a "U" each time there is a urinary leak, a "TB" each time there is a bowel movement, a "B" each time there is a bowel accident, a "G" each time there is an eight-ounce glass of fluid consumed. Indicate if it is caffeinated by an asterisk (G*), and a "P" if a new protective pad, etc., is used. Under comments, list activities and/or feelings that preceded leaks.

The second step is to summarize the bladder/bowel record results in a paragraph of five to seven sentences. Take note of the following questions in the summary.
- How often are the leaking episodes? Do they occur during one part of the day more than another? Do they occur during one type of activity more than another?

CONTINENCE PROGRAM
WEEKLY BLADDER/BOWEL RECORD

Name_____

Week of_____

INSTRUCTIONS

Insert the following symbols into the appropriate time spaces

TU = toilet urinary
TB = toilet bowel movement
U = urinary leak
B = bowel accident
G = 8oz. fluid
G* = caffeinated
P = pad

MONDAY, DATE_____
6-8 am _____
8-10 _____
10-12 _____
12-2 pm _____
2-4 _____
4-6 _____
6-8 _____
8-10 _____
10-12 _____
Overnight _____
Pads used (comments)
_____
_____

TUESDAY, DATE_____
6-8 am _____
8-10 _____
10-12 _____
12-2 pm _____
2-4 _____
4-6 _____
6-8 _____
8-10 _____
10-12 _____
Overnight _____
Pads used (comments)
_____
_____

WEDNESDAY, DATE_____
6-8 am _____
8-10 _____
10-12 _____
12-2 pm _____
2-4 _____
4-6 _____
6-8 _____
8-10 _____
10-12 _____
Overnight _____
Pads used (comments)
_____
_____

Thursday, Date_____	**Friday, Date**_____
6-8 am	6-8 am
8-10	8-10
10-12	10-12
12-2 pm	12-2 pm
2-4	2-4
4-6	4-6
6-8	6-8
8-10	8-10
10-12	10-12
Overnight	Overnight
Pads used (comments)	Pads used (comments)

Saturday, Date_____	**Sunday, Date**_____
6-8 am	6-8 am
8-10	8-10
10-12	10-12
12-2 pm	12-2 pm
2-4	2-4
4-6	4-6
6-8	6-8
8-10	8-10
10-12	10-12
Overnight	Overnight
Pads used (comments)	Pads used (comments)

- How many glasses of fluid are consumed in an average day? When is most of the fluid consumed? How much of it is caffeinated? How frequent are toileting episodes during the day, and at night?
- How many pads are used during the day, and at night? How wet is a pad when it is changed? Why is it changed?

Treatment

Once the history and bladder/bowel record summary paragraphs are combined, a much clearer picture of the incontinence story is revealed. Based on this information, decisions about medical tests can be made.

This assessment information leads to identifying the problems and appropriate treatment. Additional medical tests may be indicated with physician direction.

Treatment plans follow the Clinical Practice Guidelines of 1996, that recommend a conservative treatment trial before more invasive measures are used. Conservative treatment includes exercise, biofeedback, behavioral strategies, and medication. Health care professionals, such as nurses, physical and occupational therapists, and physicians with special training in continence exercise and biofeedback techniques, can effectively treat individuals with incontinence and develop home programs. Life style changes (see p. 63), Physiological Quieting (see p. 50), and Beyond Kegels exercises (see p. 30) are part of conservative treatment of incontinence. They can be carried out in the privacy of the home or in group exercise programs led by recreation or activity leaders.

Walking is essential to maintaining continence in the active elderly. With each step the pelvic muscle force field is activated. As the heel strikes the ground, hip external rotation occurs (obturator internus). Weight is transferred along the outer or lateral border of the foot (continued external rotation). Then internal rotation occurs (adductors/internal rotators) as weight is transferred across the transverse arch to the big toe.

Each step in walking is a pelvic muscle exercise that an individual performs without thinking about it. Twenty to thirty minutes of walking a day is therefore recommended to maintain a healthy pelvic muscle force field.

Other exercises that are derivatives of walking and benefit the pelvic muscles include:
1. Walking sideways (cruising) along a counter or railing with toes pointed outward, then toes pointed straight ahead.
2. Rotating heels together and apart in sitting or standing position.
3. Walking backwards with toes pointed outward, then straight ahead.
4. Squatting to pick up an object from the floor with the feet pointed outward.

ACTIVE ELDERLY CONTINENCE PROGRAM

Name_____ Date_____

LIFE STYLE CHANGES
❑ Caffeine Eliminated_____ cups/day
❑ Noncaffeinated Fluid/Day– 6-8 glasses
❑ Vitamin B12 (if retention)
❑ Effective Bowel Program
   Fluid___, Fiber___, Vitamin C____,
   Magnesium___, Massage___

PHYSIOLOGICAL QUIETING
Hand Warming
- Focus on warmth in your hands.
- Think to yourself, "My hands are warmer and warmer."
- "Warmth is flowing into my hands, warmer and warmer."
- Repeat 5-7 times hourly.

Diaphragmatic Breathing
- Inhale as your bellybutton rises.
- Exhale as your bellybutton falls.
- Maintain relaxed jaw, tongue, and shoulders.
- Repeat 5-7 breaths hourly.

Body/Mind Quieting
- Use *Physiological Quieting* audiotape at bedtime.

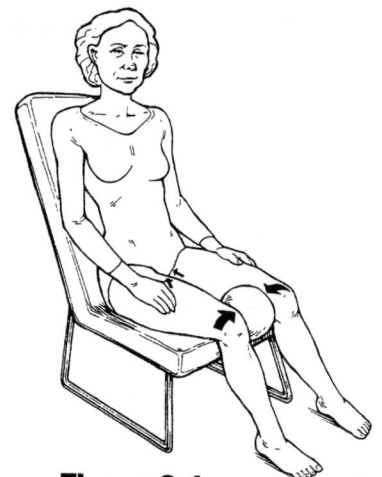

Figure 9-1

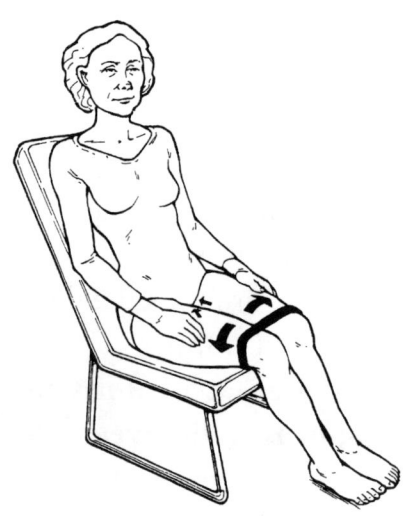

Figure 9-2

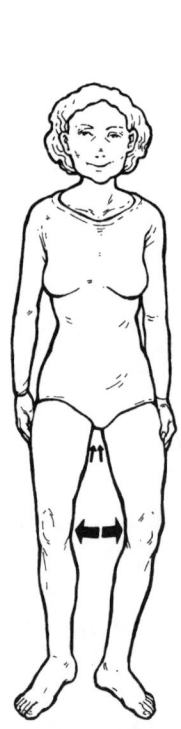

Figure 9-3

MODERATE AEROBIC ACTIVITY
- Walking is best – 20-30 minutes/day.

BEYOND KEGELS EXERCISES (5-10 Repetitions)
(Keep breathing, quiet stomach & buttocks.)
Assisted Pelvic Muscle Tightening – Adductors
(Fig. 9-1)
- Roll your knees in on Beyond Kegelball as you lift up and in with pelvic muscles.
- Hold for 10 counts, release for 10 counts.

Assisted Pelvic Muscle Tightening – Obturators
(Fig. 9-2)
- Roll your knees out against Beyond Kegelband as you lift up and in with pelvic muscles.
- Hold for 10 counts, release for 10 counts.

Standing Plíe
(Fig. 9-3)
- Stand with feet pointing outward hip width apart.
- Slowly bend knees 1-2" as you inhale for a count of 5.
- Straighten knees as you exhale, tightening pelvic muscles.
- Bend knees to a count of 5, straighten to a count of 5.
- Release/relax the pelvic muscles to a count of 5.

Urge Protocol (if needed) (see p. 73)

If UI is significant additional suggestions for treatment based on specific types of incontinence may be helpful. Further evaluation by a physician is recommended. The following outline describes treatment for stress, urge, overflow, reflex, and continuous incontinence.

STRESS INCONTINENCE
Life Style Changes:
Adequate fluid, decrease caffeine and citrus, engage in social and physical activity daily.

Smoking cessation and weight loss (both are correlated to stress incontinence).

Behavioral/Exercise Intervention:
Beyond Kegels Exercise protocol including adductor and obturator assist and quick flick exercises to develop adequate sphincteric function and improve bladder/bladder outlet position in pelvis.

Physiological Quieting protocol including hand warming and diaphragmatic breathing to normalize bladder function and autonomic nervous system innervation of bladder and bowel.

Medication Intervention:
Alpha adrenergic blockers to increase bladder outlet/sphincteric tone. Note side effects which may include headaches, insomnia, increased blood pressure.

Surgical Intervention:
Urethral suspension/support procedures and collagen injections can increase sphincteric resistance.

URGE INCONTINENCE
Life Style Change Intervention:

Adequate fluid, decrease caffeine and citrus, engage in social and physical activity daily.

Eliminate UTI and infection/inflammation by alerting physician to any signs/symptoms.

Eliminate potential bladder irritants including bubble baths, heavily chlorinated pools, perfumed toilet tissue or sanitary napkins, and artificial fiber underpants/pantyhose.

Eliminate bladder irritants including caffeine, alcohol, and aspartame. Sometimes citrus, tomato, and highly spiced foods are also bladder irritants.

Decrease urine pH by drinking cranberry juice or taking increased vitamin C which may also decrease bacterial adherence.

Increase toileting intervals to every 2-3 hours using urge inhibition if it occurs before two hour interval. Functional bladder capacity needs to be a minimum of 300cc., that often translates to 8 or more seconds of a steady urine stream.

In nursing homes answer call bells immediately, utilize bedside commode, and toilet immediately after arising from reclining.

Behavioral/Exercise Intervention:

Urge Prevention Protocol to inhibit sensation of need to void.

Beyond Kegels Exercise Protocol
Bladder Training

Medication Intervention:

Anticholinergics, smooth muscle relaxants, estrogen therapy, antibiotics.

Note: side effects of anticholinergics may include dry mouth, blurred vision, drowsiness/confusion, constipation, retention, and heat intolerance.

Surgical Intervention:

Resection or removal of tumor, lithotomy, augmentation.

OVERFLOW INCONTINENCE (RETENTION)
Medical Intervention:

Assess medications that may be decreasing bladder contractility or increasing sphincteric resistance.

Assess signs of infection, post void residual (PVR) greater than 100cc, difficulty catheterizing, trouble starting/stopping stream, hesitancy or interruption of stream, straining, or incomplete voiding.

Assess symptoms of poorly fitting pessary which could be obstructing bladder neck.

Assess bowel evacuation patterns and bowel movement consistency.

Alpha adrenergic blockers: note side effects of headache, nausea, sweating, tachycardia, hypertension, insomnia.

Clean intermittent catheterization, try not to use indwelling catheter.

Behavioral/Exercise Intervention:
　Beyond Kegels Exercise Protocol.
　Bowel Program.

Surgical Intervention:
　Suprapubic catheter, bladder pacemaker, stricture dilation, prostatectomy, anterior vaginal repair.

REFLEX INCONTINENCE
Behavioral Intervention:
　Increased cognitive awareness of voiding cue and act of voiding.
　3Ps: pants check, praise, potty.
　Timed voiding: on awakening, every 2-3 hours, prior to physical activity, after lying down, and at bedtime.

Medical Intervention:
　Assess for signs of depression.
　Assess for medication side effects increasing reflex incontinence.

CONTINUOUS INCONTINENCE
Medical Intervention:
　Rule out overflow incontinence (retention).
　Monitor PVR and notify physician if over 100cc.

Behavioral Intervention:
　Contain voids.
　Maintain skin integrity.
　Control odor.

CHAPTER 11

THE FRAIL ELDERLY
NURSING HOME AND RESIDENTIAL LIVING ENVIRONMENT

Over fifty percent of nursing home residents are incontinent. Incontinence is cited as the number two reason for admission to a nursing home. Yet, in several studies of incontinence and the elderly over 75 years of age, incontinence decreased or was eliminated with treatment. Health Care Financing Administration (HCFA) mandates bowel and bladder programs in all nursing homes, not just diapers and catheters. A comprehensive bladder and bowel continence program improves quality of life and independence. It saves dollars for the nursing home in fewer pads, sheets, and clothing used, in less disposable garbage costs, and more productive use of nursing and aide time. In some cases a continence program can facilitate a transfer for the individual to more independent living.

In the frail elderly incontinence may result from:
1. Acute or transient factors such as infection,

medications, or constipation.
2. A functional problem such as impaired mobility, manual dexterity, cognition, and/or vision.
3. Bowel and bladder system and pelvic muscle system dysfunction. The bladder, bowel and pelvic muscle systems do slow in their functioning with age but the pelvic muscles respond to stimulation much like arm and leg muscles.
4. Underlying chronic medical problems and/or use of an indwelling catheter.

Acute or Transient Factors

Incontinence may be caused by factors that are external to the bladder and bowel. Delirium, infection, medication, caffeine, restricted mobility, stool impaction, psychological factors, estrogen deficiency, or excessive urine production can lead to dysfunctional voiding. When the acute problem is solved the incontinence is resolved.

Functional Factors

The ability to independently ambulate to the toilet decreases with changes in body function. The ability to walk, to stand, and to balance decreases with arthritis joint changes, with neurological changes of aging, and with pathologies such as Parkinson's Disease. Functional mobility is impacted when muscle strength decreases due to lack of exercise and/or age. Functional endurance decreases with cardiopulmonary pathologies like COPD and emphysema.

Manual dexterity, the ability to manipulate objects with

the hands, decreases with age for many of the same reasons. In addition, manual dexterity is impacted by hand temperature. Older individuals complain of cold hands and feet. When muscles are "cold" there is decreased circulation. Cold muscles are stiff and poorly coordinated. Difficulty with zippers, buttons, and with grasping, pulling and pushing clothing increases the time needed to get on the toilet and may even prevent it without assistance.

The visual ability to locate obstacles and to locate and use the toilet is also important in maintaining continence. Other senses such as touch or hearing can be substituted to some degree but there are more episodes of incontinence when sight is limited. Incontinence increases with cognitive changes in the elderly as well. If there is decreased awareness of the need to urinate, where the appropriate place is to toilet or how to manage clothing, incontinence episodes increase.

Bowel, Bladder, and Pelvic Muscle System Dysfunction
The bladder, bowel, and pelvic muscles do slow in their functioning as an individual ages but these organs and muscles still respond to stimulation. Stress, urge, mixed, and retention types of incontinence described in previous chapters are often the results of muscle, fascia, ligaments and/or nerve dysfunction. Intervention can bring quick, effective changes in incontinence and should not be overlooked.

Underlying Medical Problems
Serious underlying medical problems may cause

incontinence. Brain injury, stroke, spinal lesions, bladder, prostate, or bowel cancers, bladder stones or hydronephrosis can lead to loss of bladder and/or bowel control. Individuals may be admitted to nursing homes with indwelling catheters because of a history of surgery, urethral blockage, coma, spinal cord injury, renal dysfunction, or intransigent incontinence.

Catheter use can be decreased with an appropriate continence program. Catheters increase patient discomfort, frequency of infections, bladder stones, and cancer. According to the Pocket Resident Assessment Protocol (RAP) Guide for the Minimum Data Set, appropriate indications for maintaining an indwelling catheter include: coma, terminal illness, stage 3 or 4 size pressure ulcer in an area affected by incontinence, untreatable urethral blockage, history of being unable to void after past catheter removal, quadriplegia or paraplegia with failed attempt to remove a catheter, or a need to measure exact urine output. Other individuals with catheters have the right to be given every chance to have them removed using a restorative program which can include Beyond Kegels exercise, prompted voiding, external catheters, or adult briefs.

ASSESS BOWEL/BLADDER INCONTINENCE

Bowel and bladder function should be evaluated within 14 days of admission as part of a total work-up of a newly admitted individual in a residential living environment. An ongoing resident should be reevaluated any time there is a significant change of status in bowel or bladder function or physical or mental ability. If changes in ability are noticed quickly, assistance or equipment can be provided to maintain continence. In the newly admitted individual appropriate protocols for treatment can be initiated as part of the daily routine. All residents should be evaluated and tracked for progress of bowel and bladder status every three months.

Other tools to detect specific characteristics of incontinence include:
1. Interview with individual and/or family to obtain history and present status (see p. 109-110 Interview Questions).
2. Interview with direct care staff to obtain current status (see p. 111-112 Staff Interview Questions).
3. Review of the medical records for medication, medical and surgical procedure history.
   If the client is catheterized the records should indicate when and why the catheter was initiated.
4. A three-day, 24 hour/day bladder/bowel record. Observe and record continence, incontinence, toileting, and verbal response to toileting prompts every two hours (see p. 113 Bladder/Bowel Monitoring Record).
5. Summarize the information from all sources on the Incontinence Master Assessment/Intervention Form (see p. 114-115).

There are several tools presently used to evaluate and track bowel and bladder continence in conjunction with other functional capabilities of the individual. Examples include the Minimum Data Set (MDS), Residential

Assessment Protocols (RAP), Functional Independence Measure (FIM), and Outcome and Assessment Information Set (OASIS). HCFA continence assessment requirements for nursing homes are contained in the MDS and RAP documents. MDS and RAPs provide assessment guidelines that facilitate an individual's optimal bladder and bowel functioning. Incontinence as a functional problem can be linked through the MDS with problems in cognition, communication, hearing, vision, mood, physical functions, structural environment, and pain. Continence in the MDS is scored on a 0 to 4 scale with 0 being continent and in complete control and 4 being multiple daily episodes of incontinence. Appliances and programs are acknowledged and integrated in the assessment. FIM assesses the level of independence or assistance needed for toileting and bladder management. The level of independence is scored from 1 to 7, 1 being minimally independent and 7 being totally independent in bowel and bladder habits. The OASIS is a mandated HCFA functional outcome assessment of daily activity items including bowel and bladder function. It is used in home health settings when an individual is homebound and receiving any rehabilitation.

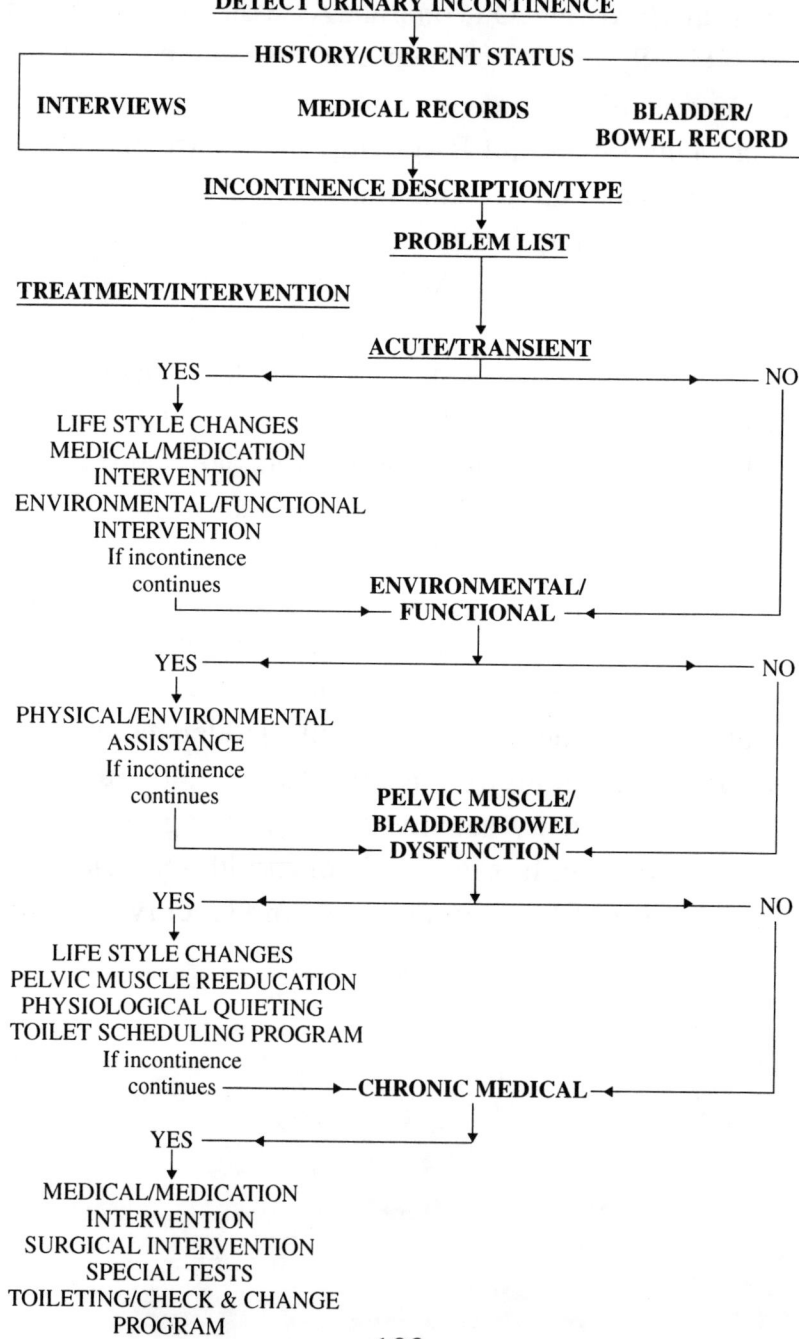

INTERVIEW QUESTIONS

Name: _____ Room # _____
Primary Informant: _____
Relation to Individual: _____

1. Describe the leaking problem. _____
2. When did the incontinence start? _____
3. What other changes occurred around this same time? _____
   _____
   (UTI, acute hospitalization, indwelling catheter, mental status change, mobility status change, surgery.)
4. Has a physician evaluated the incontinence problem? _____
   If yes, explain who and what was done, i.e. history, physical exam, urinalysis/culture, cystoscopy, urologic consultation, etc.) _____
   _____
   _____
5. Has there been any previous treatment for urinary problems? ____
   If yes, what? _____
   _____
   If treated, what was the response to treatment? _____
   _____
6. Is an indwelling catheter used? ____yes ____no
   If yes, date initiated _____ Reason_____
7. What if anything is currently being used to manage leaking?
   tissue paper or pads ____   special undergarment ____
   bed pad at night   ____   medication   ____ list_____
   schedule voiding   ____   _____
   external catheter   ____   limit fluids   ____
   other_____ _____
8. What is the pattern of urination during the day?/night?

	every 30 min.	1-2 hours	3-4 hours
Day	_____	_____	_____
Night	_____	_____	_____

9. Are there any difficulties during urination?
   difficulty starting the flow ____   slow, dribbling stream ____
   straining to finish toileting ____   pain or discomfort   ____
   urge/frequency   ____   dribbling after urination ____
10. What is used during urination (U)? What is used during bowel movements (BM)?

	day	night
bathroom commode	___	___
bedside commode	___	___
urinal	___	___
bedpan	___	___
diaper/padding	___	___
external catheter	___	___

11. Is it physically possible to use the toilet or toilet substitute
    without help?   ____Yes   ____No
    If no, what is the limitation?_____
    Rate the ability to perform the following:

	independent	needs assist	total assist
transport self to toilet	____	____	____
transfer to toilet	____	____	____
manage clothing	____	____	____
position urinal/bedpan	____	____	____
clean self after toileting	____	____	____

12. How frequent are incontinent episodes?
    ____weekly   ____1xday   ____2-3xday   ____more
13. Is incontinence during day or night or both?   ____day   ____night   ____both
14. What is the volume of urine lost?
    ____small (less than 1/4 cup)   ____large (1/2 cup or more)   ____variable
    Explain:_____
15. Leaking occurs when:
    ____individual has no urge to toilet during the day
    ____during the night while asleep
    ____individual expresses need then leaks
    ____coughing, sneezing, laughing
    ____changing in position from sit to stand or supine to sit, or walking
16. Is there awareness...   ____when bladder is full?   ____when urine is flowing?
    Is there request to toilet...____when bladder is full?   ____when urine is flowing?
17. What color is the urine?_____Is there an odor to the urine?
    ____Yes   ____No   Describe:_____
18. How many cups of fluid are consumed each day? _____   # caffeinated____
    What fluids are preferred?_____
19. List all medication presently used. _____
    _____
    _____

20. Has there been any skin breakdown?   ____Yes   ____No
    Describe: _____ _____
    What skin care products are being used? _____
21. What is mental status?   ____alert/responsive   ____disoriented/forgetful
                              ____cooperative   ____uncooperative
22. What is communication status?   ____verbal communication   ____aphasic
    ____poor comprehension   ____slow comprehension   ____good comprehension
23. What is vision status?   ____adequate   ____needs aid (glasses, etc.)
                              ____poor   ____blind
24. What is hearing status?   ____adequate   ____needs aid   ____poor   ____deaf

Summarize on Incontinence Master Assessment/Intervention Form (p.114).

STAFF INTERVIEW QUESTIONS

To ask the Licensed Staff Nurse:
1. Is this resident interviewable?
2. How much assistance does the resident require in the activities of daily living?
3. Was the resident continent when he/she was first admitted? When was that?
4. Why is the resident incontinent? *(Cause)*
5. How did you determine reasons for resident's incontinence?
   (How were assessed-tests done?)
6. Can the problem be treated? Is the incontinence reversible?
   (If applicable) Why did you decide not to apply treatment program?
7. What are the risk factors related to this resident's care needs?
8. What are you presently doing to assist the resident in managing the incontinence?
9. How effective is the treatment?
10. What other staff disciplines are involved in assisting this resident to be dry?
11. To be asked if resident has a catheter:
    a. When did the resident get the catheter?
    b. Was he/she admitted with the catheter in place?
    c. Do you know why he/she has a catheter? Was any other intervention tried before the catheter?
    d. How long will the resident need a catheter?

    e. Has the resident experienced any urinary tract infections?
    f. Has the resident been given a voiding trial? What happened?
    g. How is the catheter care given?

To ask the direct care staff aide:
1. When did the resident first become incontinent, if you know?
2. How often do you find the resident wet?
3. What do you do when the resident is wet?
4. How do you know what to do when the resident is wet?

To ask the resident:
1. Would you mind talking with me about your toileting and how you manage?
2. When did you first have this problem?
3. Was that before or after you came to live here?
4. Why do you think you have this problem? Did your doctor or nurse talk with you about it?
5. Use History form if appropriate.

BLADDER/BOWEL MONITORING RECORD

Record date, initial box for each shift. Check individual every two hours and record findings.
Record three-day baseline data.

DATE	INITIAL													CODE					# OF PADS	# OF VERBAL RESPONSES	COMMENTS
		7-3			3-11			11-7													
		7am	9	11	1pm	3	5	7	9	11	1am	3	5								
Day 1																					
Day 2																					
Day 3																					

SUMMARY (# From Above)

DATE	U	B	★	TU	TB	T	X	Pads	VC
Day 1									
Day 2									
Day 3									
TOTAL									
% OF TOTAL TRIALS (36)									

CODES: EVERY TWO HOURS

U – Episode of Urinary Incontinence
B – Episode of Bowel Incontinence
★ – Clean and Dry
TU – Independent or Assisted to Toilet - Urinated
TB – Independent or Assisted to Toilet - Bowel Movement
T – Assisted to Toilet - No Result
X – Not Cooperating
PADS – / = 1 pad used
+ / – Response to Verbal Cue (VC)
"Are you wet or dry?"

INCONTINENCE MASTER ASSESSMENT/INTERVENTION FORM

Name_____ Rm #_____

Asses. Date	Problem Yes	Problem No	Reason for Incontinence	Intervention Date	No Change	Incontinence % Improve	Ceases
			ACUTE / TRANSIENT REASONS				
			1. Urinary Tract Infection				
			2. Atrophic Urethritis / Vaginitis				
			3. Stool Impaction / Constipation				
			4. Caffeine / Alcohol				
			5. Delirium				
			6. Psychological (Depression)				
			7. Increased Urine Production (High Blood Calcium or Glucose)				
			8. Other				
			MEDICATION REASONS				
			1. Diuretics				
			2. Sedations				
			3. Antidepressants				
			4. Antipsychotics				
			5. Antihistimines				
			6. Antispasmodics				
			7. Phenothiazines				
			8. Over the Counter				
			9. Other				
			ENVIRONMENTAL / FUNCTIONAL REASONS				
			1. Bed / Chair Transfers				
			2. Toilet / Chair Transfers				
			3. Standing Balance / Sitting Balance				

Continued ☛

Name_____

Eval. Date	Problem Yes	Problem No	Reason for Incontinence	Intervention Date	No Change	Incontinence % Improve	Incontinence Ceases
			ENVIRONMENTAL / FUNCTIONAL REASONS				
			4. Dressing / Clothing				
			5. Personal Hygiene After Toileting				
			6. Range of Motion – Functional				
			7. Mode of Locomotion				
			8. Vision				
			9. Hearing				
			10. Mental Awareness / Cooperation				
			11. Lower Extremity Edema				
			12. Manual Dexterity				
			13. Other				
			BLADDER / PELVIC MUSCLE REASONS				
			1. Stess Incontinence				
			2. Urge Incontinence				
			3. Mixed Incontinence				
			4. Overflow Incontinence				
			5. Nonrelaxing Puborectalis				
			6. Other (Fecal)				
			MEDICAL REASONS				
			1. Endocrine / Metabolic (Diabetes, Thyroidism)				
			2. Cardiac / Circulation				
			3. Pulmonary (COPD)				
			4. Neurologic – Brain Dysfunction				
			5. Neurologic – Spinal Cord				
			6. Orthopedic – Fracture / Replacement				

Continued ☛

Name_____

Eval. Date	Problem Yes	Problem No	Reason for Incontinence	Intervention Date	No Change	Incontinence % Improve	Ceases
			MEDICAL REASONS				
			7. Orthopedic – Amputation				
			8. Arthritis – Rheumatoid / Osteoarthritis				
			9. Psychiatric				
			10. Cancer				
			11. Renal Failure				
			12. Other				
			SUMMARY OF 3-DAY MONITORING RECORD				
Comments	Day 1	Day 2	Day 3	Total			
# Leaks/Day							
# Leaks/Night							
# Pads/Day							
# Hrs/Dry/Day							
# Hrs/Dry/Night							
# Toileting Successes							
# + Verbal Prompts							
# BMs/DAY							

SUMMARY PROBLEM LIST

ACUTE/TRANSIENT
1. _____
2. _____
3. _____

MEDICATION
1. _____
2. _____
3. _____

ENVIRONMENTAL/FUNCTIONAL
1. _____
2. _____
3. _____

BLADDER/PELVIC MUSCLE
1. _____
2. _____
3. _____

MEDICAL
1. _____
2. _____
3. _____

Signature_____ Date_____

RECOMMENDATIONS FOR INCONTINENCE INTERVENTION PROGRAM

Name _____

Note: Pelvic muscle reeducation program is carried out concurrently with any other program.

☐ 1. **ACUTE/TRANSIENT PROGRAM**
   - The goal is to eliminate or minimize acute/transient problems that cause incontinence including bowel impaction/constipation.
   - Appropriate to intervene with this first.
   - These factors may preclude success in other incontinence programs.

☐ 2. **ENVIRONMENTAL/FUNCTIONAL ASSIST PROGRAM**
   - The goal is to provide physical/verbal/environmental assistance to promote independent bladder and bowel control.
   - Appropriate if incontinence increased due to environmental or physical limitations.

☐ 3. **PELVIC MUSCLE REEDUCATION PROGRAM**
   - The goal is to improve independent bowel/bladder function and improve continence.
   - Appropriate if individual can roll hips in and out with verbal or touch prompts.
   - Indwelling catheter, UTI must be eliminated first. Monitor medical recommendations before beginning this program.

☐ 4. **BLADDER/BOWEL SCHEDULING PROGRAM**
   - The goal is to schedule/prompt assistance to maintain continence at present or better level when unable to do so alone.
   - Appropriate if individual is dry or urinates in toilet more than 50% of the time and responds to verbal prompts more than 50% of the time.

☐ 5. **CHECK AND CHANGE PROGRAM**
   - The goal is to check individual for wetness every two hours, reposition and change garments when wet/soiled.
   - Appropriate if unresponsive to verbal prompts and unable to toilet consistently.

☐ 6. **Refer to physician for medical problems.**

Reassess on _____ for possible change in program.

_____   _____
Signature   Signature

BLADDER/BOWEL INTERVENTION PROTOCOL

Instructions: Check module, fill in dates of intervention and of improvements.

Initial Intervention	Intervention Dates	Incontinence No Change	% Improve	Ceases
☐ **ACUTE/TRANSIENT PROGRAM** 1. Urinary Tract Infection - Antibiotics 2. Hypoestrogenation - Estrogen 3. Other Comments:				
☐ **BOWEL PROGRAM** (3 weeks) 1. Nutritional Changes – Fluids 2. Nutritional Changes – Foods 3. Nutritional Changes – Magnesium, Vit. C 4. Bowel Habit Program 5. Other Comments:				
☐ **PELVIC MUSCLE REEDUCATION PROGRAM** 1. Beyond Kegels Exercises - Easy Active (3 weeks) 2. Beyond Kegels Exercises - Easy Resistive (3 weeks) 3. Other Comments:				
☐ **ENVIRONMENTAL/FUNCTIONAL ASSISTANCE PROGRAM** (3 weeks) 1. Environmental Changes 2. Transfers Modification 3. Locomotion Modification 4. Personal Hygiene 5. Vision, Hearing, Communication 6. Mental Awareness 7. Other Comments:				
☐ **MEDICAL/MEDICATION PROGRAM** 1. Medication Changes 2. Medical Condition Intervention 3. Other				
☐ **SCHEDULING/CHECK & CHANGE PROGRAM** 1. Prompted Voiding 2. Scheduled Voiding 3. Check and Change Comments:				

Name_____ Rm#_____

RESULTS SUMMARY – BLADDER/BOWEL TRAINING

Instructions: Add three day total and divide by three.

3-Day 2-Hr. Check	Baseline	Bowel	Beyond Kegel Easy-Active	Beyond Kegel Easy-Resistive	Other
# Leaks / Day					
# Leaks / Night					
# Pads / Day					
# Hrs Dry / Day					
# Hrs Dry / Night					
# Toileting Successes					
# BMS/DAY					

Comments:

Note: Program Intervention Time Line: 3-days baseline, 3-day reassessment recorded at end of each 3 week protocol. 3 weeks for each category: bowel protocol, BK Exercises – Easy Active, BK Exercises – Easy Resistive.

RESULTS SUMMARY – PROBLEM LIST

Instructions: Fill in date resolved, % change and no change.

PROBLEMS	INCONTINENCE		
	Resolved	% Change	No Change
ACUTE/TRANSIENT 1. 2. 3.			
ENVIRONMENTAL/FUNCTIONAL 1. 2. 3.			
PELVIC MUSCLE DYSFUNCTION 1. 2. 3.			
MEDICAL/MEDICATION 1. 2. 3.			

Summary Description_____

Signature_____ Date_____

IDENTIFY POTENTIAL REASONS FOR INCONTINENCE

From the interviews, history, bladder/bowel diary, and medical records review, identify potential reasons for incontinence and categorize on the Incontinence Master Assessment/Intervention Form (see p. 114). The reasons are divided into problem categories which include:
1. Transient/Acute Caused Problems.
2. Environmental/Functional Problems.
3. Bladder/Bowel/Pelvic Muscle System Problems.
4. Chronic Medical Problems.

TRANSIENT/ACUTE PROBLEMS INCLUDE:
Urinary Tract Infection (UTI)

Dysuria and urgency from a UTI may defeat the ability to reach the toilet in time.

Atrophic Urethritis or Vaginitis

Hypoestrogenism causes atrophic changes in genitourinary and pelvic muscle systems. Dysuria, dyspareunia, burning during urination, and urgency are common symptoms.

Stool Impaction

Bowel dysfunction leads to urge, stress, and overflow bladder incontinence.

Diuretics

The bladder is overwhelmed with fluid leading to polyuria, frequency, and urge incontinence. Diuretics increase severity of present incontinence.

Caffeine

Caffeine acts as a diuretic. It is also a bladder muscle irritant and a nervous system irritant. Frequency, urge, and stress incontinence may occur.

Other Medications

Anticholinergic agents can lead to urinary retention, frequency, overflow and functional incontinence.

Sedatives, hypnotics, CNS depressants, alcohol accumulate in the elderly and can cause confusion and impaired mobility leading to functional incontinence.

Alpha-adrenergic agents such as antihistamines, sympathomimetics (decongestants) and sympatholytics can induce retention and overflow incontinence.

Calcium channel blockers reduce smooth muscle contractility causing retention and overflow incontinence.

Delirium

Incontinence is often an associated symptom.

Psychological

The relationship between psychological conditions and incontinence is not completely understood but is present.

Restricted Mobility

Limited mobility secondary to an acute or chronic illness or injury (arthritis, poor eyesight, Parkinson's disease, stroke) leads to functional incontinence.

Increased Urine Production

Hyperglycemia, hypercalcemia lead to excessive fluid intake, then diuresis, and possible incontinence. Excessive fluid intake or volume overload from venous insufficiency with edema or congestive heart failure can lead to incontinence.

ENVIRONMENTAL/FUNCTIONAL PROBLEMS INCLUDE:

Instances when the individual is aware of the need to toilet (without urgency), but can't get to or use the toilet include:
1. Physical limitations including manual dexterity,
2. Inappropriate clothing,
3. Cognitive limitations, confusion, or disorientation (medications may be implicated),
4. An unfamiliar environment,
5. Inaccessible or inadequate facilities,
6. Vision limitations,
7. Hearing limitations,
8. Pain, and
9. Lack of privacy.

To determine functional/environmental problems assess the living environment and physical, mental, and sensory capabilities of the individual.

Assistive devices can be essential for an individual to be continent. Assistive devices may be an intermittent catheter, a urinal, a bedpan, or a bedside commode. A more independent individual may be continent with use of a wheelchair, walker or cane, a raised or lowered toilet seat, arm and/or back support for the toilet, or support bars on the bathroom walls. If manual dexterity is an issue, clothing alteration including elastic waistbands and velcro fasteners can increase the speed of clothing removal.

The potti test assesses the time needed for manual tasks related to toileting (Ouslander et al. 1987). Those tasks include:
1. Moving 15 feet to the toilet.
2. Transferring to a commode.
3. Unfastening a hook and unzipping a zipper.
4. Removing an apron or gown.

The individual is placed 15 feet from the toilet with an apron-like garment containing a zipper and hook or button on it. The individual is instructed to get to the toilet, then to sit on the toilet, then to unzip and unbutton the zipper and button or snap, and finally to remove the garment. If the individual can complete all tasks in approximately 60-99 seconds continence is usually possible. If it takes over 100 seconds prompted voiding procedures may need to be initiated.

Toilet hygiene independence is also important to assess. This includes tearing off toilet paper, use of toilet paper or wet wipes to clean, including grasping the item and moving it from front to back to clean the perineal area. Reach to buttocks for cleaning after a bowel movement is assessed. If needed, assessment for assistive toilet aids or tongs and methods of use is completed.

The level of assistance needed for continence varies

from independent to maximal assistance. Assistance includes supervision (standing by, cueing, encouraging), set up of equipment (placing or emptying devices), or transfer assistance on and off the toilet. Transfer assistance may vary from assistance with positioning and locking the wheelchair to one or two persons assisting transfer from wheelchair to toilet. The extent of assistance available and practical will vary with the environment the individual lives in (Schnelle, 1991).

If the individual is in bed the majority of the day ask if the individual can:
1. Grasp the urinal or bedpan?
2. Place the urinal or bedpan in position?
3. Remove the urinal or bedpan?

If the individual is in a wheelchair the majority of the day ask if the individual can:
1. Wheel self to commode or bathroom?
2. Transfer from chair to commode or toilet?
3. Transfer from toilet to chair?
4. Clean self?
5. Remove clothing?

If the individual uses a bedpan or urinal ask the questions for individuals in bed.

If the individual is independent or uses a cane or walker ask if the individual can:
1. Get up from the chair?
2. Get up from the bed?
3. Walk to the toilet or commode?
4. Rise from the commode or toilet?

5. Remove clothing?
6. Clean self?

Aids, assistance, and training is provided when deficits are noted.

It is possible to be continent without being ambulatory, but it takes more planning and assistance.

In addition to physical assistance the individual must have cognitive skills to attain continence. In severe dementia and late stage Alzheimer's disease, low level of cognitive functioning may preclude independent continence even though physical skills remain high. Screen for cognitive skills by asking the following questions:

1. "Are you wet or dry?"
2. "Show me the bathroom."

If the individual cannot show you the path to the bathroom he/she will need staff prompts to maintain continence. A large picture of a toilet, a large print word "toilet" taped on the outside of the bathroom door, or painting the door a bright color may be an adequate prompt. If the individual does not respond at all to the question "Are you wet or dry?" there is inadequate cognitive processing or motivation to be independently continent. If the individual responds but with the wrong answer it is appropriate to initiate a trial continence program. Prompted voiding can help compensate for cognitive problems.

BLADDER/BOWEL/PELVIC MUSCLE SYSTEM PROBLEMS INCLUDE:
1. **Stress Incontinence**
2. **Urge Incontinence**
3. **Mixed Incontinence**
4. **Fecal Incontinence/Constipation**

In **Stress Incontinence** the individual is unable to hold urine when intra-abdominal pressure increases. This may be caused by an underactive urethra, decreased bladder outlet resistance, an unstable urethra, or genuine stress urinary incontinence (GSUI). In females, decreased pelvic muscle tone and/or estrogen depletion leading to atrophic vaginitis/urethritis can lead to stress incontinence. In males, urethral damage following radical prostatectomy and reduced urethral closure pressure from medication use (alpha adrenergic blockers) are the most common causes.

The individual will present with loss of urine with coughing, sneezing, laughing, getting up from sitting or lying down, bending, pushing, pulling.

In **Urge Incontinence** the individual is unable to inhibit voiding when the sensation to void is present. This may be caused by detrusor instability, hyperreflexia, overactive, uninhibited, or unstable bladder. In males and females causes include bladder tumors or stones, high volume voids secondary to diuretics or excessive intake, urinary tract infection, inflammation, radiation therapy, concentrated urine, or limited functional bladder capacity. In females, estrogen deficiency leading to atrophic vaginitis/urethritis may cause urge incontinence.

The individual presents with the awareness of an urgent need to void but not enough lead time to get to the toilet.

In **Mixed Incontinence** the individual exhibits a combination of stress and urge symptoms with a combination of causes.

In **Fecal Incontinence/Constipation** the individual is unable to have a bowel movement two or more times per week and/or experiences periodic diarrhea. Abdominal discomfort may also be a factor.

CHRONIC MEDICAL PROBLEMS INCLUDE:
1. **Reflex Incontinence**
2. **Continuous Incontinence**
3. **Overflow Incontinence**

Serious medical problems can include brain or spinal cord lesions, bladder or prostate cancer, renal failure, heart or pulmonary conditions, diabetes, or other endocrine dysfunctions or musculoskeletal problems.

Types of incontinence resulting from serious medical problems include Reflex Incontinence, Continuous Incontinence, and Overflow Incontinence.

In **Reflex Incontinence,** the individual is unable to inhibit voiding because sensation is absent. Possible causes include diseases, injuries, or neurologic disorder interfering with communication between the brain and bladder; delirium (medications may be implicated–analgesics or tranquilizers); CVA or stroke; dementia; demyelinating diseases; peripheral nerve lesions; trauma; and severe mental retardation.

The individual presents with loss of urine but no awareness of the leaking.

In **Continuous Incontinence,** the individual is unable to hold any urine. The individual presents with constant dribbling of urine. Possible structural damage to urethra post surgery, post radical prostatectomy, hysterectomy, or bladder augmentation may be the cause.

In **Overflow Incontinence,** the individual is unable to void and completely empty bladder. This may be caused by an atonic, flaccid neuropathic, paralytic, or underactive bladder. Possible causes include decreased bladder contractility, neurologic disease, surgery, pharmacotherapy (anticholinergics, psychotropics, antiparkinsonians, antispasmodics, opiates, Beta adrenergic blockers) or chronic overdistention. Other causes may be urethral obstruction from stricture, enlarged prostate, cystocele, or stool impaction. Increased sphincteric resistance from pharmacotherapy (antihistamines, alpha adrenergic stimulants) or obstructive atrophic vaginitis/urethritis (from postmenopausal estrogen deficiency) can cause retention and overflow.

The individual presents with toileting frequently in small amounts and may be continent or incontinent.

Serious medical problems need to be referred for medical workup unless it has already been done.

INITIATE TREATMENT FOR INCONTINENCE

When the results of assessment indicate an incontinence problem, a continence program/voiding trial is indicated. A problem exists when:
1. Incontinence occurs two or more times per week.
2. Use of external (condom) catheter, indwelling catheter, or intermittent catheter is present.
3. Use of pad or briefs is ongoing.

Treatment progresses from the most simple to the more complex. Treatment can be as simple as eliminating coffee or as complicated as a surgical procedure.

Treatment progresses from:
1. Eliminating transient/acute problems to
2. Addressing environmental/functional problems to
3. Addressing bladder/bowel/pelvic muscle dysfunction to
4. Understanding bladder/bowel toileting program and/or
5. A check and change program to
6. Physician referral for chronic medical problems.

Initiate treatment to eliminate the transient/acute problems first. Then reassess the individual's incontinence status (see p. 114 for appropriate record forms).

Treat **functional/environmental problems and bladder/bowel/pelvic muscle dysfunction** next. These can be run concurrently at times. See Recommendations for Incontinence Intervention Programs and Bladder/Bowel Intervention Protocol (see p. 117, 118).

TREATMENT STRATEGIES FOR TRANSIENT/ACUTE PROBLEMS INCLUDE:

Problem	Intervention Strategy
Urinary Tract Infection	Antibiotics, fluids
Atrophic Urethritis, Vaginitis (Hypoestrogenation)	Vaginal estrogen cream, Hormone replacement therapy
Stool Impaction, Constipation	Reduce impaction, Bowel program (see p. 26)
Diuretics	Change schedule/dosage Change diuretic
Caffeine Intake	Eliminate coffee, tea chocolate, pop/soda
Other Medications	Physician directed change of medication Pharmacist consult
Delirium	Physician directed treatment
Psychological	Physician directed treatment of depression, paranoia, etc.
Restricted Mobility, Restricted Manual Dexterity	Physical assistance, Assistive devices, Adaptive clothing (see Functional/Environmental Treatment)
Increased Urine Production	Physician directed treatment

TREATMENT FOR FUNCTIONAL/ ENVIRONMENTAL INCONTINENCE INCLUDES:

Medical Intervention

Reverse confusion and disorientation by alerting M.D. to medications that may cause altered states.

Arrange pain medication schedules that allow comfortable ambulation and sitting.

Life Style Change Intervention

Reverse confusion and disorientation by systematically reorienting confused individuals.

Tape the word "toilet" or picture of toilet on outside of bathroom door at eye level for wheel chair use.

Improve toilet accessibility and visibility.

1. Use siderails and restraints only when medical symptoms indicate.
2. Keep beds in low positions.
3. Choose chairs which are easy to get out of.

Provide adequate, nonglaring lighting.

Leave bedside commodes and urinals close at hand.

Leave mobility aides (wheelchairs, walkers, crutches, canes) and eyeglasses close at hand.

Provide easy access to call buttons.

Provide assistance to toilet, bedpan, urinal, or bedside commode.

Use elevated seats and grab bars for patients having difficulty getting down or up from regular toilets. Individualize toilet selection.

Assure privacy with closed doors and pull curtains as well as appropriate clothing.

Institute communication system for nonverbal patients.

Improvise back support and foot rests to give optimal support.

Use elastic waist pants in place of zippers and buttons.

Behavioral/Exercise Intervention

PT/OT assessment to evaluate strength, mobility, footwear, clothing, toilet seating.

Functional exercises of toileting movement patterns broken down into small components.

Reinforce use of handrails, safety belts, assistive devices.

TREATMENT TO ELIMINATE BLADDER/BOWEL/PELVIC MUSCLE SYSTEM PROBLEMS INCLUDES:

1. A Bowel Program

The goals are to have regular bowel movements and eliminate constipation and stool impaction. Nutrition, exercise and a bowel habit protocol are components of the bowel program (see p.26 and 119 for detailed procedures).

2. Pelvic Muscle Reeducation

The goal is to improve function of the pelvic muscles in support of the bladder and bowel, and in control of urine and feces continence. Reeducation implies improved muscle coordination with other muscles, improved nerve/muscle/brain function, as well as improved muscle strength. It is a coordination issue as much or more than a strength issue (see Chapter 2, Anatomy/Physiology).

The exercises include:
1. Beyond Kegels – easy active.
2. Beyond Kegels – easy resistive.
3. Standing Plíe.

PATIENT EDUCATION TOOL
MUSCLES THAT AID IN BLADDER CONTROL – HOW THEY WORK

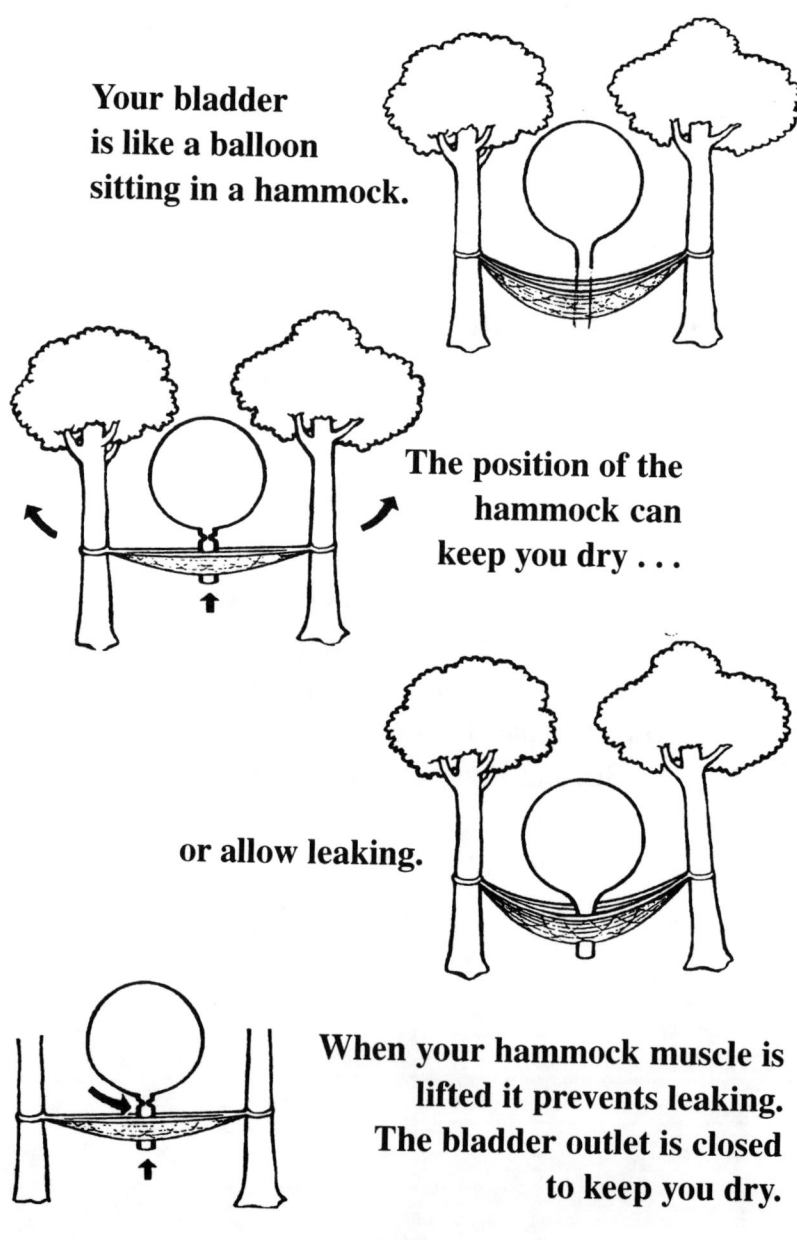

Your bladder is like a balloon sitting in a hammock.

The position of the hammock can keep you dry . . .

or allow leaking.

When your hammock muscle is lifted it prevents leaking. The bladder outlet is closed to keep you dry.

BEYOND KEGELS – EASY, ACTIVE EXERCISES

To lift your hammock muscle – roll your knees apart then bring them back together. This helps strengthen the hammock muscle and prevent leaking.

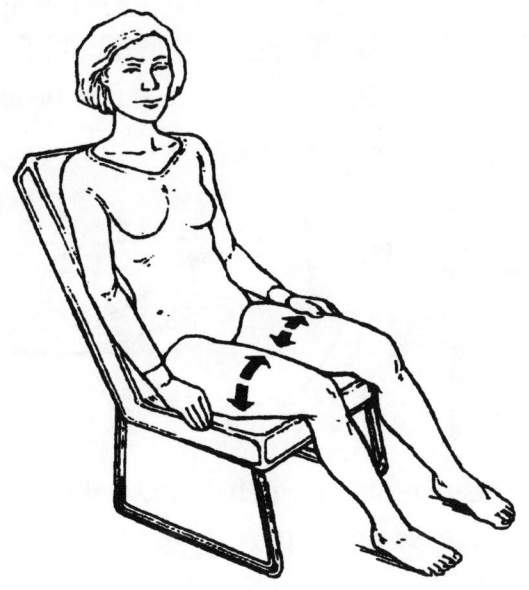

In the morning, in the middle of the day, and in the evening . . . roll your knees out and roll them in – 10 repetitions. You can do it in a sitting position or lying down.

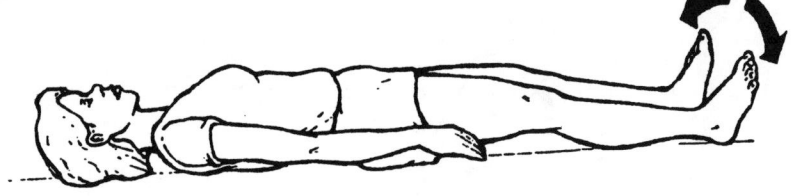

BEYOND KEGELS – EASY, RESISTIVE EXERCISES

When the exercises are easy you can add some resistance.

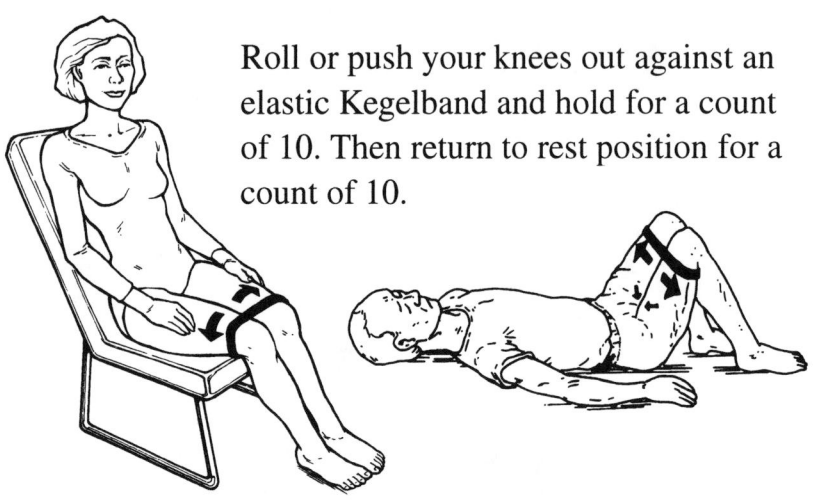

Roll or push your knees out against an elastic Kegelband and hold for a count of 10. Then return to rest position for a count of 10.

Roll your knees in on a Kegelball and hold for a count of 10. Then release pressure coming to neutral to rest for a count of 10.

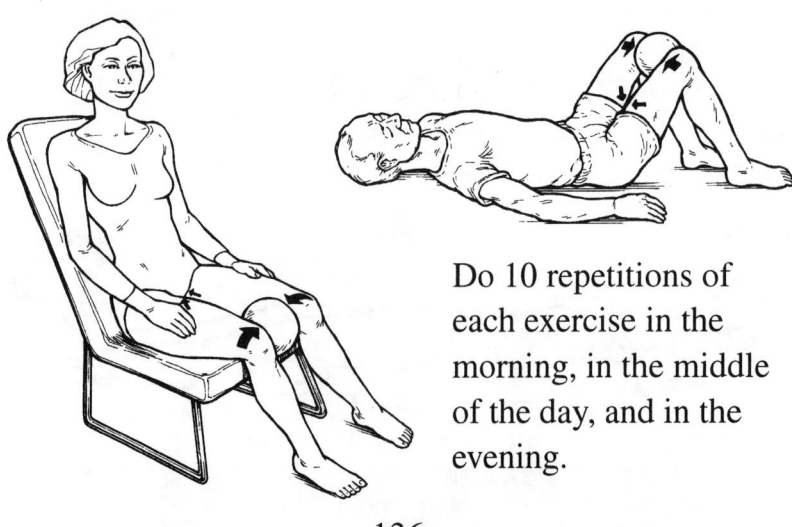

Do 10 repetitions of each exercise in the morning, in the middle of the day, and in the evening.

BEYOND KEGELS – STANDING PLÍE

When the previous exercise is easy, and if you can be in a standing position, add one more exercise.

Stand with your back against a wall and with your toes pointing out like a duck. Hold on to a chair if needed.

Slowly bend your knees 1-2 inches, then straighten them. Do 5-10 repetitions a day.

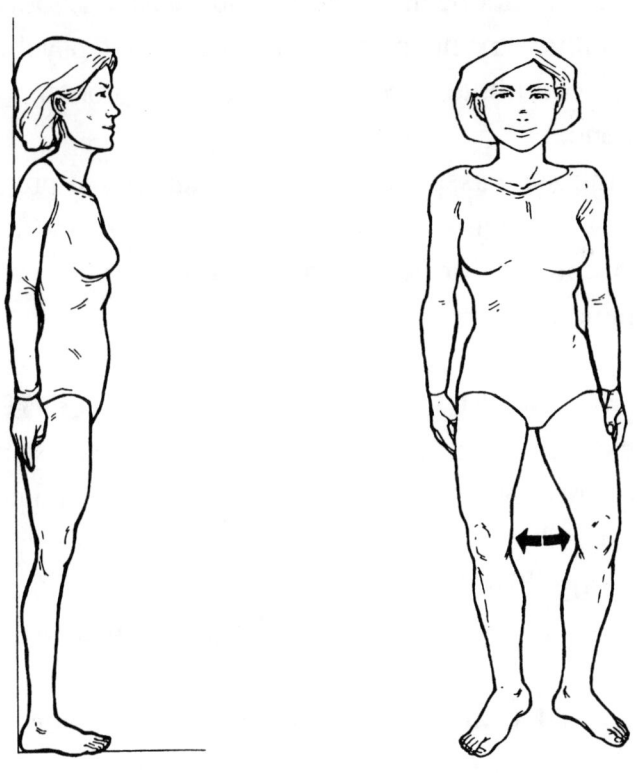

TREATMENT FOR CHRONIC MEDICAL PROBLEMS

Physician directed medical intervention includes advanced tests, i.e. urodynamic testing, medications, and surgery, among others. Urodynamic testing is appropriate at times to help determine pathologies and possible surgery. Medications for medical conditions or medication changes are important to monitor on a regular basis. Surgery to repair structures may be indicated and can significantly impact bladder and bowel control.

Medical intervention for chronic medical problems which lead to secondary incontinence is appropriate if these problems have not been previously addressed. Endocrine, cardiac, pulmonary, neurologic, orthopedic, and psychiatric conditions contribute directly or indirectly to problems with incontinence.

Continuous reassessment is important to see progress and/or new problems. Quarterly assessment of continence status in conjunction with other functional outcomes is recommended.

BLADDER/BOWEL SCHEDULING TREATMENT

Assessment criteria can indicate toileting management protocols are appropriate. Toileting management and pelvic muscle reeducation programs most often are run concurrently. Toileting management protocols include scheduled toileting, prompted voiding, and timed voiding.

Scheduled voiding involves setting a predetermined interval for voiding assistance, for example every two hours. This is easier in the institutional setting than timed voiding and does not involve as much time for assessment of personal intervals. It involves no verbal prompting.

Prompted voiding is scheduled voiding with verbal prompting and reinforcement included. This technique is preferred since it has the advantage of reducing passivity and facilitating more independence. It takes no more time than scheduled toileting after the initial training .

Prompted voiding involves five steps according to Schnelle. They are check, talk, prompt, praise, and correct.

Check involves changing the individual's position and doing a physical check for wetness.

Talk involves asking the individual "Are you wet or dry?" up to three times and giving accurate feedback to the individual.

Prompt involves asking the individual if they will try to use the toilet or other device. The question is repeated up to three times in a persuasive manner. The individual is never toileted unless he/she answers in the affirmative.

Praise involves positive feedback for:
1. Making an effort to use the toilet.
2. For being dry. Statements like "Very nice Ms. Jones, you are dry."

Correction involves giving an appropriate corrective statement if the individual is wet. Statements like, "You are wet Ms. Jones, please tell me before you have to go next time." If the individual is wet but tries to use the toilet give praise but no correction.

Timed voiding involves discovering the individual's intervals between voidings and/or leaking and assisting them to the toilet just prior to these times. The interval can be difficult to determine and may change frequently. In an institutional setting it is difficult to remember many individual schedules.

CHECK AND CHANGE MANAGEMENT TREATMENT

Check and change protocol involves an aide physically checking the individual every two hours for wetness, and if wet, changing the undergarment and repositioning the individual. Night time check and change periods can often be extended to 3-4 hours if the individual exhibits increased dry periods.

ASSESS NEED FOR TOILETING OR CHANGING TREATMENT

The **three day bladder/bowel monitoring record** is the basis for determining whether a toileting or check and changing protocol is most appropriate. Over the span of three days, every two hours data is kept on toileting, urine leaks, and verbal responsiveness. If the individual gives no verbal or nonverbal response when asked every two hours "Are you wet or dry?" the individual must be placed on a check and change protocol. It is not necessary for the individual to speak clearly, rather nodding or other hand or body movements indicating wet or dry are acceptable. It is not necessary for the individual to give a correct response, rather the importance is that he/she responds at all. The question should be repeated up to three times before concluding the individual has no response. This question is one of the most valid mental response screens to determine suitability for a toileting or exercise program.

In addition, to be successful in a prompted voiding toileting program, the individual must be able to:
1. Start the voiding process if given access to a toilet.
2. Hold urine during intervals between toiletings.

If the verbal responsiveness is positive the next step is to assess the ability to void when on the toilet and hold urine between toiletings. If the individual toilets or is dry greater than fifty percent of the two hour trials and responds greater than fifty percent to the wet/dry questions, he/she is a good candidate for a prompted voiding trial. Even if the data doesn't indicate a high prediction for total continence many individuals will show a major improvement in volume of urine leaked and/or the frequency of leaking when the Beyond Kegels exercise protocol and prompted voiding are used together.

Summarize the results of treatment on a regular basis – every three weeks if active intervention is occurring. Record dates and results on the Bladder/Bowel Intervention Protocol form (see p. 118). For research purposes and required for HCFA documentation, a three day bladder/bowel monitoring record is done at the end of each intervention category (see p. 114). For example, a three day record would be collected after 3 weeks of the bowel protocol, after 3 weeks of the pelvic muscle reeducation protocol, and after 3 weeks of prompted voiding.

CHAPTER 12

TOTAL HIP REPLACEMENT, HIP FRACTURE AND INCONTINENCE

TOTAL HIP REPLACEMENT/HIP FRACTURE

Incontinence and hip fracture/total hip replacement are frequent companions in the elderly. Incontinence can be a key risk factor for falling and hip fracture. The question is as yet unanswered as to the potential increase in incontinence after total hip replacement/hip fracture repair procedures. Incontinence and hip fracture are major reasons for nursing home admissions.

Thousands of individuals experience hip fractures each year. When there is hip replacement surgery, the obturator internus is avulsed from the greater trochanter. In some surgical procedures there is an attempt to reattach the obturator, in others the obturator is left to find it's own attachment. Even when the obturator is reattached, a significant number of attachments fail to take. The function of the obturator internus in supporting the bladder and bowel through the pelvic muscle force field can therefore be compromised in an asymmetrical way.

Additionally, during surgery there is the potential for damage to nerves and nerve plexuses that innvervate the pelvic muscles, bladder, and bowel. Functionally, the individual's mobility to get to the bathroom is significantly affected after hip fracture/surgery and catheterization is often routine. Emotionally, there may be some depression and/or disorientation from the fall, the surgery, and the change in living environment. All of these factors can precipitate long term loss of bladder/bowel control or exacerbation of previous dysfunction.

To prevent and/or alleviate the incontinence associated with hip fracture/total hip replacement it is essential to incorporate pelvic muscle exercises with the total hip protocol exercises already being done.

The following are examples of hip protocol exercises with incorporation of pelvic muscle exercises. The combination means that incontinence can be prevented and/or eliminated in individuals with total hip/hip fracture utilizing one group of exercises. If incontinence remains a significant problem the addition of the Beyond Kegels exercises and Physiological Quieting is recommended.

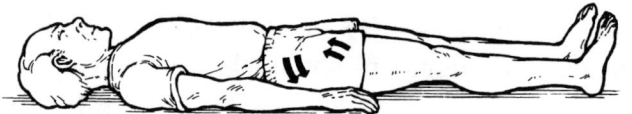

Figure 12-1

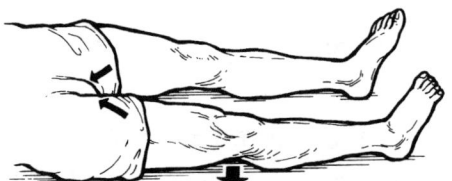

Figure 12-2

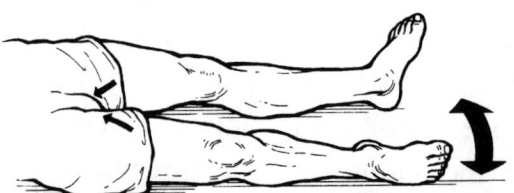

Figure 12-3

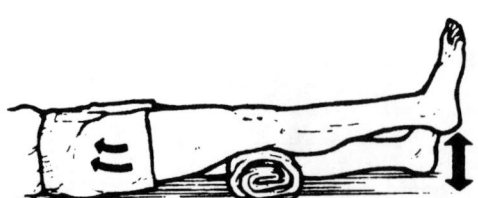

Figure 12-4

HIP REPLACEMENT/HIP FRACTURE

In supine, maintain diaphragmatic breathing during all exercises.

Repeat each exercise 5-10 times.

1. **Gluteal Sets** (In supine, sitting, or standing.) (Fig. 12-1)
   - Lift the pelvic muscles up and in.
   - Simultaneously tighten the buttocks muscles.
   - Hold for a count of 5 and release for a count of 5.

2. **Quadriceps Sets** (Fig. 12-2)
   - Lift the pelvic muscles up and in.
   - Simultaneously tighten the quadriceps, pushing the knee(s) into supporting surface.
   - Hold for a count of 5 and release for a count of 5.

3. **Hip Rotation** (Fig. 12-3)
   - Lift the pelvic muscles up and in.
   - Simultaneously roll the toes out so they point toward the side wall.
   - Return to neutral position, toes pointing to the ceiling.
   - Roll out for a count of 5, roll in to neutral for a count of 5. Rest for a count of 5.

4. **Short Arc Quads** (Fig. 12-4)
   - Lift the pelvic muscles up and in.
   - Simultaneously straighten the knee with the heel off the ground.
   - Hold for a count of 5 and release for a count of 5.

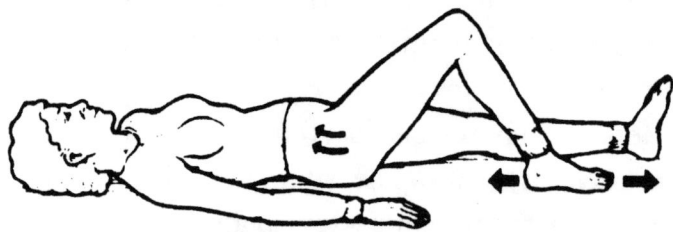

Figure 12-5

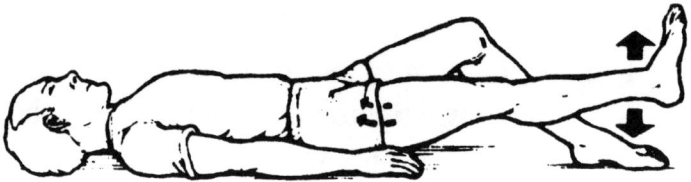

Figure 12-6

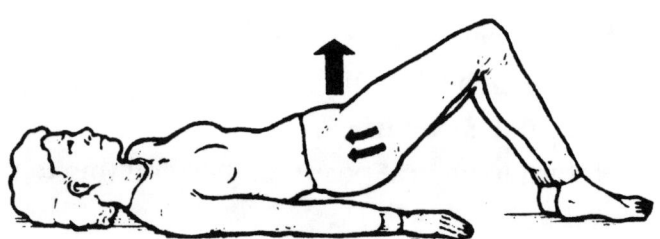

Figure 12-7

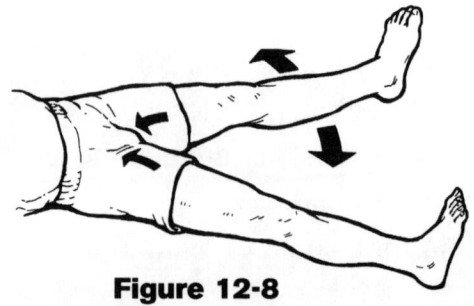

Figure 12-8

5. **Heel Slides** (Fig. 12-5) Supine.
    - Lift the pelvic muscles up and in.
    - Simultaneously slide the heel slowly towards buttocks.
    - Increase the knee bend while keeping hip flexion <90°.
    - Slide for a five count, return for a count of 5, rest for a count of 5.

6. **Straight Leg Raises** (Fig. 12-6) Supine, 1 leg flexed.
    - Lift the pelvic muscles up and in.
    - Lock the knee and lift the foot about 12" off the bed.
    - Hold for a count of 5 and return to the rest position.

7. **Hip Bridges** (Fig. 12-7) Hooklying.
    - Lift the pelvic muscles up and in.
    - Tighten abdominal and buttocks muscles gently.
    - Lift the buttocks off the bed, keeping pelvis level.
    - Hold for a count of 5, return to rest position for a count of 5

8. **Hip Abduction** (Fig. 12-8) Supine.
    - Lift the pelvic muscles up and in.
    - Simultaneously slide the involved leg out then in.
    - Slide for a count of 5 in, count of 5 out, and rest for a count of 5.

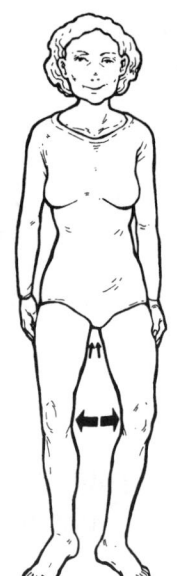

Figure 12-9

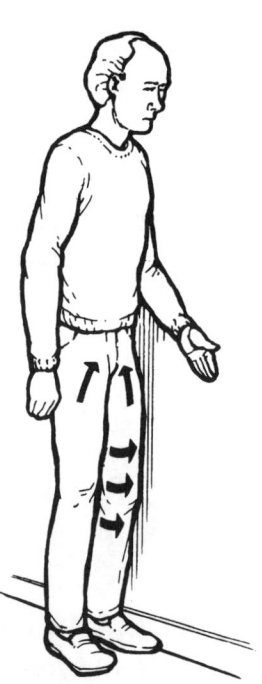

Figure 12-10

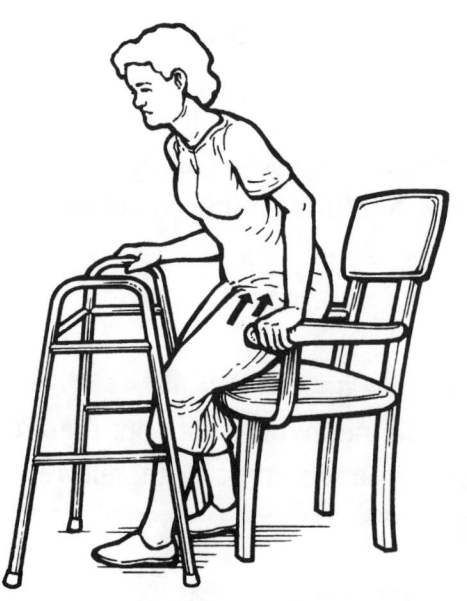

Figure 12-11

Standing Plíe (Fig. 12-9) Standing position.
- Stand with feet pointing outward, hip width apart.
- Slowly bend knees 1-2" as you inhale for a count of 5.
- Straighten knees as you exhale, tightening the pelvic muscles.
- Release/relax the pelvic muscles to a count of 5.
- Bend knees for a count of 5, straighten for a count of 5, relax for a count of 5.

Standing Isometric Lateral Rotation (Fig. 12-10)
In standing position with the affected leg touching the wall.
- Focus on slow, low diaphragmatic breathing.
- Roll knee out against wall while lifting pelvic muscles up/in.
- Hold for a count of 5. Then release for a count of 5.
- Repeat 5-10 times.

Sit to Stand (Fig. 12-11)
- Place affected foot ahead of unaffected foot with toes pointed out.
- Place one hand on arm of chair, one hand on handgrip of walker.
- Focus on slow, low diaphragmatic breathing.
- Lean head forward over knees.
- Lift up and in with the pelvic muscles.
- Simultaneously push up to a standing position.

CHAPTER 13

FOR MEN ONLY
BENIGN PROSTATE HYPERPLASIA
ERECTILE DYSFUNCTION-IMPOTENCE
RADICAL PROSTATECTOMY

Incontinence problems in men often begin after 65 years of age. Men experience hormonal changes after 50 but do not have the same amplitude of changes as women. From 40 on, however, the prostate gland gradually enlarges in response to changes in the levels of testosterone. This enlargement may lead to leaking during exertion, urge sensations, frequency of urination, incomplete emptying

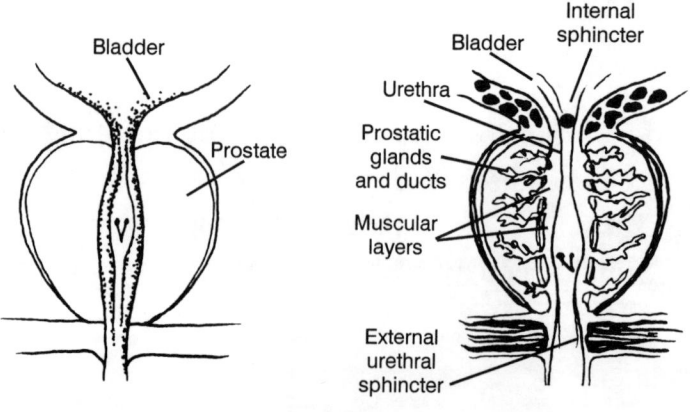

of the bladder, and/or weak urine flow. As the prostate enlarges it narrows the proximal urethra at the bladder outlet which increases resistance to urine flow from the bladder through the urethra. Bladder (detrusor) muscle contractile efficiency decreases with age and hormonal changes so it does not push urine down the urethra as effectively.

Men do not usually experience incontinence problems earlier because there are several effective anatomical mechanisms that prevent leaking. Between the bladder outlet and the prostate gland, at the proximal end of the urethra, is the internal sphincter muscle that automatically contracts or closes to keep urine in the bladder and relaxes to release urine. At a more distal end of the urethra, below the prostate gland, are the external sphincter and urogenital diaphragm muscles which are under voluntary control and assist in control of urine. The prostate gland and urethra have smooth muscle layers which contract to stop urine flow and relax/release to facilitate flow of urine outward.

Benign Prostate Hyperplasia

As the prostate enlarges, it can occlude or block the urethra so urine cannot flow out effectively and efficiently, even though the bladder may be contracting to push the urine out and the internal and external sphincter muscles are relaxed to release urine. Symptoms of this obstruction can include:
1. A weak stream of urine.
2. Frequent feelings of urge to urinate but only small amounts of urine are released.

3. Relatively small leaks of urine during physical activity.
4. Occasional large leaking episodes when there is the urge to toilet and it has been several hours since the last toileting and /or a considerable fluid intake.

Urethral blockage by the prostate gland can cause incomplete emptying of the bladder. Post void residual (PVR), the urine left in the bladder after toileting, can be excessive (greater than 100cc) and lead to:
1. Bladder lining irritation.
2. Bladder infection.
3. Urine reflux into the kidneys.
4. Depression from depletion of vitamin B12.

Prostate enlargement can be benign/nonmalignant or cancerous. If it is benign, a transurethral prostatectomy (TURP) can be performed to remove the excess tissue that is blocking the urethra. It is termed by some the "roto rooter" method of treating the prostate problem. A long tube is place through the urethra and into the bladder. Like a cystoscope, the miniature camera within the tube can inspect the urethra and bladder. When the excess prostate tissue is located, another device is used through the tube to remove the tissue. The surgery takes about one hour and the individual may be in the hospital 2-3 days. A rare, but occasional, result of this surgery can be total or partial urinary incontinence.

Erectile Dysfunction–Impotence

Erectile dysfunction (ED), also termed impotence, is the inability to achieve or maintain an erection sufficient for satisfactory sexual performance. Partial or total ED is experienced by as many as 30 million men. Fifteen to twenty-five percent of men over 65 years old experience ED. Diabetes, vascular disease, surgery including radical prostatectomy, multiple sclerosis, endocrine dysfunction and psychosocial factors may lead to ED.

Treatment includes prosthetic implantation of flexible rods/inflatable devices, vascular reconstruction, medications, vacuum tumescence, psychotherapy, and therapeutic exercise.

Perineal muscle exercises can help return forty to fifty percent of men with ED to satisfactory sexual function if nerve innervation and circulation are intact. The urogenital diaphragm muscle contractions increase intracavernous pressure and coincide with increased penile rigidity as intracavernous pressure exceeds systolic blood pressure. The corpora is compressed by the ischiocavernosus muscle of the urogenital diaphragm and becomes closed chambers. Blood, as incompressible fluid, flows to the uncompressed portion of the corpora expanding the envelope, increasing intracavernous pressure resulting in an erection.

Beyond Kegels roll in and out and quick contraction exercises are beneficial in treating erectile dysfunction when nerve innervation and circulation is intact (see Chapter 5).

Radical Prostatectomy

In cancerous enlargement of the prostate gland, radical prostatectomy surgery is often recommended. There is complete removal of the prostate gland and related tissue in the hope of eliminating all cancerous cells. The internal sphincter and urethra contained in the prostate are removed in the procedure. In some cases, pelvic lymph nodes are also removed. Other treatment options such as chemotherapy, radiation therapy, and hormonal therapy including removal of the testicles to eliminate testosterone, may be used either alone or in conjunction with radical prostatectomy.

The possible sequal of radical prostatectomy, radiation, chemotherapy, and/or hormonal therapy include incontinence, detrusor instability with small bladder capacity, erectile dysfunction and denervation of the pudendal nerve. After these procedures as many as one third of men may experience incontinence or frequency a year after surgery. An even greater percentage experience erectile dysfunction.

Questions to ask men having incontinence problems after a radical prostatectomy include:
1. Are you able to void in the toilet?
2. Are you able to start urine flow easily?
3. Is the urine stream strong or weak?
4. Do you have an urge to void sensation, ie. Do you know when its time urinate?
5. Is there pain or burning during urination?
6. Are you able to stop the urine flow completely at the end of urination?

7. Do you leak with a strong urge, with movement, with coughing or sneezing?
8. How many pads do you use during the day/night and how wet are they?
9. How frequently do you toilet during the day, at night?
10. How much fluid are you drinking each day and what kind?

The answers to these questions can lead to appropriate treatment to minimize incontinence. If an individual is unable to void, overflow incontinence and/or obstruction may be the problem. Eliminating the obstruction is recommended. Intermittent catheterization is often used to maintain normal PVR. If there is continuous urine flow months after the surgery, then stove pipe urethra is often the diagnosis. An artificial sphincter is one solution to this problem. If urine flow is difficult to initiate or the flow is weak there may be a non-relaxing puborectalis muscle, a stricture, or decreased bladder contractions. Exercise, biofeedback, and medication are all treatment options to relax the pelvic musculature and improve detrusor contraction strength. If the urge to void sensation is absent it may indicate bladder overdistension or impaired contractions. Pain or burning during voiding indicates a possible infection and medication is the treatment of choice. Dribbling after the completion of urinating indicates dysfunction of the external urethral sphincter or detrusor instability (excessive bladder contractions). Exercise and physiological quieting are often effective if innervation is intact.

Knowing the type of incontinence and the amount of leaking assists in prioritizing a treatment protocol. Stress incontinence treatment will emphasize different exercises and medications than urge incontinence.

TREATMENT
Treatment–Nutrition

One of the first actions taken by men experiencing urinary incontinence of any nature is to decrease fluid intake throughout the day and night. While the immediate result of this may be a little less leaking, the long term results can be devastating. Less fluid in the bladder causes the bladder to shrink. The bladder responds to the volume of liquid by adjusting in size, much like a balloon that enlarges as it is filled with air and shrinks when that air is released. A smaller bladder often results in more leaking. A smaller bladder sends more frequent messages to the brain that it has to empty. Eventually the individual may be toileting every 30 minutes during the day and hourly at night.

The decrease in urine also causes serious problems. Less urine means the urine is more concentrated and may irritate the bladder lining. This can cause the bladder to contract more frequently and strongly. Some men describe it as an explosion of urine they cannot control. Concentrated urine can lead to bladder and lower abdominal discomfort and even bladder infections.

It is important that 6-8 glasses of noncaffeinated fluid be consumed daily. It is appropriate to stop fluids after

6:00 p.m. to facilitate longer periods between toileting during the night. The fluid intake is best if it is spread out evenly through the day.

The herb saw palmetto and the mineral zinc, 25-30mg, may be helpful in the treatment of incontinence secondary to benign prostate hyperplasia. Vitamin B12 injections/supplements are often recommended for men with incontinence, as well. Vitamin B12 is important to supplement because it can be significantly depleted with urine retention (high PVR) and this depletion can lead to depression.

Treatment–Bowel Protocol

With aging, and particularly after prostate surgery men have bowel concerns. Constipation exacerbates urinary incontinence. Excessive pushing can cause bleeding from the surgical site. A bowel program is recommended for most men (see p. 26).

Treatment–Urge Protocol

It is important for the elderly to know the techniques to use when the feeling of urge occurs but when there has not been at least 2 hours since the last toileting (see p. 73).

Life Style Change Intervention:

Maintain social and physical activity daily.

Eliminate UTI by alerting physician to any signs/symptoms.

Eliminate bladder irritants including caffeine, alcohol, and aspertame. Sometimes citrus, tomato, and highly spiced foods are also bladder irritants.

Decrease urine pH by drinking cranberry juice or taking increased vitamin C which can decrease bacterial adherence. Taking antioxidants with bioflavoroids decreases the pH without all the sugar.

Increase toileting intervals to every 2-3 hours using urge inhibition protocol if it occurs before 2 hour interval. Functional bladder capacity needs to be a minimum of 300 cc. or an 8-12 second stream of urine.

In nursing homes, answer call bells immediately, utilize bedside commode, and toilet immediately after reclining.

Treatment–Physiological Quieting (PQ)

There is a tendency for men who experience leaking to tighten every muscle in the pelvic area in an attempt to stop the involuntary flow of urine. They tighten the buttocks, pelvic muscles, external anal sphincter, and abdominal muscles in a chronic maximal contraction. These muscles eventually fatigue and thus even more leaking occurs. The first step in treatment for most men is learning how to completely relax these muscles. Start the individual with body/mind quieting, then progress to specific muscle quieting (see p.50).

Treatment–Beyond Kegels Exercises

The next step in treatment is learning to submaximally contract/tighten only the appropriate muscles, while leaving the others relaxed. Contraction of the appropriate muscles–the pelvic diaphragm, urogenital diaphragm, and external sphincter muscles in conjunction with the obturator internus–is the goal. The third step is to practice repetitions that gently contract and then completely relax this pelvic muscle force field. The fourth step is to increase the contraction intensity, continuing to alternate equal contraction and relaxation periods (see p. 160, 161).

Standing exercises are important, too. The standing plíe is easy to do and repetitions can be dispersed throughout the day (see p. 160, 161).

Men often orient the pelvic muscle contraction to the anal area rather than the urethral or penis portion of the muscular hammock. To orient the contractions towards the urethral area, have the individual place his hands on the lower abdomen/symphysis pubis area and contract towards the finger tips. Another technique involves contraction of the pelvic muscles to make the penis move up and down a quarter to one-half inch. Exhaling forcefully through pursed lips, as when blowing out a lot of candles, can also help recruit more anterior fibers.

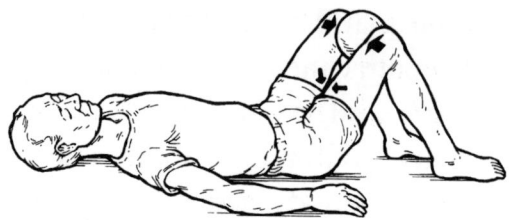

Figure 13-1

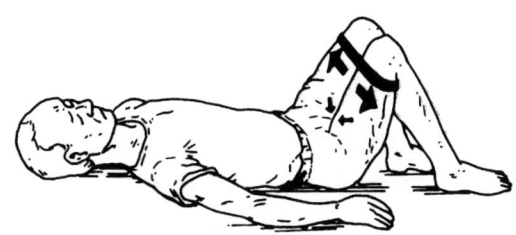

Figure 13-2

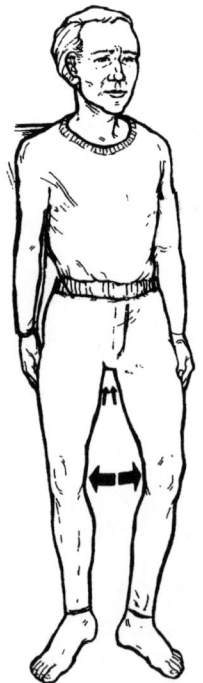

Figure 13-3

ASSISTED PELVIC MUSCLE TIGHTENING
Roll In – Using Adductors (Fig. 13-1)

Position for this exercise is reclined on the bed or floor with hips and knees bent and feet resting flat on the supporting surface. Place a Beyond Kegelball between the knees. Roll your knees in on the ball and tighten the pelvic muscles as if you were going to stop a bowel movement. Hold while counting out loud to 10. Then relax your knees and pelvic muscles and rest for a count of 10.

Roll Out – Using Obturator Internus (Fig. 13-2)

Position for this exercise is reclined on the bed or floor with hips and knees bent and feet resting on the supporting surface. With knees together tie a Beyond Kegelband around the legs just above the knees. Roll your knees out against the elastic band and tighten the pelvic muscles as if you were going to stop a bowel movement. Hold while counting out loud to 10. Then relax your knees and pelvic muscles and rest for a count of 10.

Standing Plíe (Fig. 13-3)

Stand with feet pointing outward hip width apart. Slowly bend knees 1-2" as you inhale for a count of 5. Straighten knees as you exhale, tightening the pelvic muscles. Bend knees to a count of 5, straighten to a count of 5. Release/relax the pelvic muscles to a count of 5.

CHAPTER 14

PROTECTIVE PRODUCTS FOR INCONTINENCE

Incontinence products are used to absorb lost urine or leaks. They enable the individual to lead a more active, complete life without the fear of odor or wetness. No single product will work for all individuals or in every circumstance. Exploring all options and having several types of products on hand enables the fullest, most spontaneous life style. Incontinence products can be purchased at pharmacies, grocery stores, or through mail order companies (see Resources p. 165).

Considerations in choosing incontinence products should include absorbency level, size, fit, comfort, disposability, changeability, and cost. If loss of urine is small at any one time then light, thin pads that attach to underwear will be adequate. If leaks are large and/or constant then a super absorbent, larger product is needed. If night time leaking is a problem, bed pads and absorbent underwear pads may both be necessary.

The appropriate incontinence product will comfortably

fit the contours of the body to prevent leaking outside the protection, yet not chafe or cut off circulation. It will be invisible with no lines or folds visible through outside clothing. The ease of changing and disposal of incontinence products is important. When manual dexterity or balance in sitting or standing is limited, ease of application and removal will be a priority. The cost of the product may determine if the individual purchases and uses it.

Absorbent pads and adult diapers/briefs are the two major categories of protective products for the elderly. Absorbent pads come in many sizes and absorbency levels– from small, light pads to super absorbent, larger pads. Pads with self adhesive tape attach to regular underwear, slip into pockets in special underwear, or attach to a belt. Pouch-like pads for men are available. They fit around the penis and/or scrotum and fasten to the underwear. Adult diapers or briefs tape, button, or snap around the hips/waist. They can be disposable or reusable. Elastic legs and super absorbent material turns liquid into gel to prevent leakage.

EXAMPLES OF INCONTINENCE PROTECTION

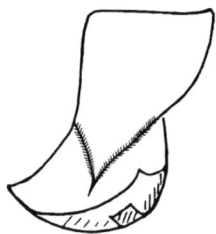 Disposable Pads for mild to moderate leakage.

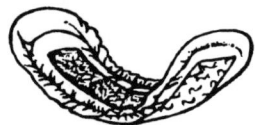

Disposable pouches for men with mild to moderate leakage.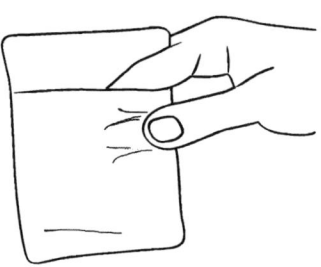

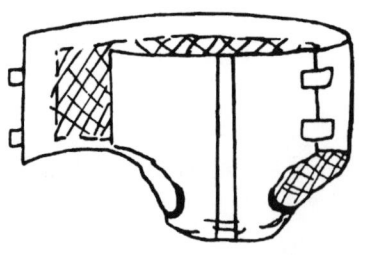 Disposable briefs for full bladder containment.

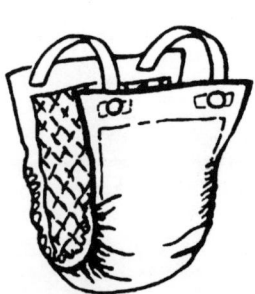

RESOURCES

National Association for Continence (NAFC)
   P.O. Box 8310
   Spartenburg, SC 29305-8310
   1-800-BLADDER
   Introductory information packet, quarterly newsletter, highlights from industry – new products

International Foundation for Functional Gastrointestinal Disorders
   P.O. Box 17864
   Milwaukee, WI 53217
   1-888-964-2001
   Newsletter, publications, symposiums

InContiNet – internet site
   http://www.InContiNet.com

National Institute of Diabetes and Digestive and Kidney Diseases – National Institute of Health
   3 Information Way
   Bethesda, MD 20892-3580
   1-800-891-5388
   Educational resource guide, publications

The Simon Foundation for Continence
  P.O. Box 815
  Wilmette, IL 60091
  1-800-237-4666

US, TOO International, Inc.
  930 North York Rd., Ste. 50
  Hinsdale, IL 60521
  Prostate cancer/disease support group

Society of Urologic Nurses and Associates (SUNA)
  East Holly Ave.
  Box 56
  Pitman, NJ 08071-0056
  1-609-256-2333

Wound, Ostomy, and Continence Nurses (WOCN)
  2755 Bristol St., Ste. 110
  Costa Mesa, CA 92626

American Urological Association (AUA)
  P.O. Box 7600
  Wilkes-Barre, PA 18773-7600
  1-713-665-7500

Women's Health Section – American Physical Therapy Association
  P.O. Box 327
  Alexandria, VA 22313
  1-800-999-2782 Ext. 3387

Health Care Financial Administration (HCFA)
   6325 Security Blvd. BPD
   E. High Rise Bldg., Rm. 489
   Baltimore, MD 21207

A+ Medical Products, Inc.
   16 Alden Place
   Newton, MA 02165
   1-888-843-3334
   Female catheter guide, female urinal

Kimberly-Clark Corporation
   2001 Marathon Ave.
   Neenah, WI 54957-9002
   1-800-558-6423
   Educational material, protective products

Home Delivery Incontinent Supplies, Inc. (HDIS)
   1215 Dillman Industrial Court
   Olivette, MO 63132
   1-800-269-4663
   Protective products and supplies

REFERENCES

Beyond Kegels: Fabulous Four Exercises and More ... To Prevent and Treat Incontinence. Janet A. Hulme. Missoula, MT: Phoenix Publishing, 1997.

Beyond Kegels Book II: A Clinician's Guide To Treatment Algorithms & Special Populations. Janet A. Hulme. Missoula, MT: Phoenix Publishing, 1998.

Biofeedback, 2nd Edition. Mark S. Schwartz and Associates. New York: The Gilford Press, 1995.

Clinical, Functional, and Psychosocial Characteristics of an Incontinent Nursing Home Population. Ouslander, J.G., et. al. Journal of Gerontology, 42(6), 631-637, 1987.

Constipation: Etiology, Evaluation & Management. Steven D. Wexner and David C.C. Bartolo. Oxford: Butterworth-Heinemann, Ltd., 1995.

Everyone Poops. Taro Gomi. Brooklyn: Kane/Miller Book Publishers, 1993.

Female Urology, 2nd Edition. Schlomo Raz. Philadelphia: W.B. Saunders Company, 1996.

Fibromyalgia: A Handbook for Self Care & Treatment, 2nd Edition. Janet A. Hulme. Missoula, MT: Phoenix Publishing, 1997.

Fundamentals of Anorectal Surgery. David E. Beck and Steven D. Wexner. New York: McGraw-Hill, Inc., 1992.

Guide for the Uniform Data Set for Medical Rehabilitation – Section III: Functional Independence Measure (FIM Instruments) UB Foundation Activities, Inc., 1996.

Let's Get Things Moving: Overcoming Constipation. Pauline Chiarelli and Sue Markwell. Health Books, 427/150 Queen St., Woolahra NSW 2025, Australia (contact National Association for Continence)

Managing Urinary Incontinence in the Elderly. John F. Schnelle. New York: Springer Publishing, 1991.

Minimum Data Set for Nursing Home Resident Assessment and Care Screening. Natick, M.A.: Eliot Press.

Nursing for Continence. Katherine F. Jeter, Nancy Faller and Christine Norton. Philadelphia: W.B. Saunders, 1990.

Outcome Assessment (OASIS), Outcome Based Quality Improvement. Shaughnessy, P. & Creslor, K. National Association for Home Care, 1995.

Pocket Rap Guide for the Minimum Data Set V2. Natick, M.A.: Eliot Press, 1995. 1-508-655-8123.

Staying Dry: A Practical Guide to Bladder Control. Kathryn Burgio, Lynette Pearce and Angelo Lucco. Baltimore: The Johns Hopkins University Press, 1989.

Topics in Clinical Urology: Evaluation and Treatment of Urinary Incontinence. Jerry Blaivas, New York: Igaku-Shoin, Inc., 1996.

The Honest Herbal. V.E. Tyler. New York: Haworth Press, 1993.

Urinary Incontinence. Pat O'Donnell. St. Louis: Mosby-Year Book, Inc., 1997.

Urinary Incontinence in Adults: Clinical Practice Guideline. AHCPR Publication No. 92-0038. Rockville, MA: Agency for Health Care Policy and Research, Public Health Service, U.S. Dept. of Health and Human Services, 1996.

Urologic Nursing: Principle and Practice. Karen Karlowicz. Philadelphia: W.B. Saunders Co., 1995.

GLOSSARY

Anal Sphincter Two rings of muscles surrounding the rectum and anus which help to control passage of bowel movements.

Anus Muscular opening at the end of the rectum is the outlet for solid waste.

Behavior Therapy Treatment involving conditioning.

Benign Prostatic Hyperplasia (BPH) Condition characterized by growth of a benign tumor inside the prostate, often resulting in voiding difficulties. Also known as benign prostate hypertrophy.

Benign Tumor Noncancerous tissue growth that cannot spread to other areas of the body.

Biopsy Diagnostic procedure of surgically removing a tissue sample from the body and analyzing it microscopically for abnormal tissue growth.

Bladder Muscular organ located inside the pelvis for temporary storage of urine.

Blood Count Test used to determine the number and ratio of red and white blood cells and platelets in an individual's blood. Abnormal numbers can indicate infection, anemia, or cancer.

Blood Tests Samples of individual's blood that can include a blood count, sedimentation rate, glucose level, cholesterol and triglyceride levels, and special tests for prostate cancer (PSA and PAP tests).

Bulbocavernous Muscle One of three muscles of the urogenital diaphragm.

Cancer Disease characterized by uncontrolled cell growth and spread of cells to other parts of the body. Cell growth can crowd out or interfere with normal cell function causing organ dysfunction and death of healthy cells.

Castration Removal of testes or elimination of testicular function with antiandrogen drugs.

Catheter Flexible tube inserted into a body part such as the urethra (in male or female) to empty the bladder of urine.

Cervix Lower portion of the uterus that connects with the vagina.

Chemotherapy Cancer treatment using potent drugs that attack and destroy tissue cells and interfere with the cells multiplying. These drugs are either injected or taken orally.

Clitoris Organ of female orgasm.

Collagen Chemical substance injected into the internal urinary sphincter region to treat incontinence.

Colon Lower portion of large intestine leading to the rectum.

Computerized Tomography (**CT scan**) A computer-enhanced X-ray technique used to examine soft body tissue,

Congestion Buildup of fluid in an area of the body that often causes pain, i.e., prostate congestion.

Constipation Hard, dry, and firm bowel movements that are difficult to pass and less frequent than normal.

Contraindication Side effects of a medical treatment which would indicate the treatment is more harmful than the intended benefits.

Cryosurgery Surgery that utilizes extreme cold to destroy undesired tissue.

Cystocele Bulging of the bladder into the anterior vaginal wall.

Cystogram Tube with light and a viewing lens at the end, which is inserted into the urethra to examine the urethra, bladder, and prostate gland.

Cystoscopy Diagnostic procedure for urological examination allowing viewing inside the urethra and bladder.

Diagnosis Determination through observation or scientific tests of the existence of symptoms of medical disorders.

Diuretic Any drug, food, or beverage that promotes increased urine excretion.

Encopresis Uncontrolled passage of bowel movement or smears of fecal material into underwear or inappropriate places by an individual over the age of four.

Enterocele A bulging of the pouch of Douglas into the posterior vaginal wall.

Enuresis Involuntary loss of urine, during sleep termed "nocturnal."

Episiotomy Surgical incision into the perineum between the vagina and anus to ease childbirth through the vagina.

Estrogen Hormone contributing to female sex characteristics, produced in female ovaries and male testicles, in adrenal glands, and fat.

Functional Incontinence Physical disability or mental confusion leading to inability to void in an appropriate place.

Hormone Chemical substances made in endocrine glands and essential for human biological processes.

Hormonal Therapy Treatment based on administering hormone or chemical substances that block the action of other hormones. Hormonal therapy blocks action of male hormones that promote tumor growth.

Hysterectomy Surgical removal of the uterus.

Iliococcygeal Muscle One of the muscles forming the pelvic diaphragm/levator ani muscle group.

Impotence Inability of a man to achieve or maintain an erection of sufficient duration.

Incontinence Loss of urinary control.

Intravenous Pyelogram (IVP) Diagnostic procedure to examine the urinary system with X-ray after injecting image-enhancing substances into the bloodstream.

Introitus The external vaginal opening.

Ischiocavernous Muscle One of three muscles forming the urogenital diaphragm.

Ischiococcygeal Muscle Also known as the puborectalis muscle, one of the three muscles forming the pelvic diaphragm/ levator ani muscle group.

Kegel Exercises Pelvic muscle exercise to decrease or eliminate incontinence.

Kidneys Two glandular organs that separate waste products from the blood.

Magnetic Resonance Imaging (MRI) Diagnostic technique using an electromagnetic field and computer analysis, which effectively evaluates soft body tissue, such as the prostate and bladder.

Menopause Cessation of menstruation, usually occurs in the late 40's or early 50's.

Orchiectomy Surgical removal of testicles.

Overflow Incontinence Temporary inability to void, followed by uncontrollable urine flow, associated with overdistension of the bladder.

Pelvic Diaphragm The levator ani muscle group.

Pelvic Muscles General term referring to the muscles of the pelvic diaphragm and urogenital diaphragm as one unit, sometimes referred to as the pelvic floor muscles.

Penis The male organ used for urination.

Perineum/Perineal Muscles Area of muscle and tissue between the vagina or scrotum and anus.

Prostate Firm, muscular gland that surrounds the urethra in males.

Prostatectomy Surgical removal of all or part of the prostate gland.

Prostatitis Infection of the prostate; can be acute or chronic.

Pubic Bone Lower front part of the pelvis.

Pubic Symphysis Where the two pubic bones meet.

Pubococcygeal Muscle One of three muscles forming the pelvic diaphragm/levator ani muscle group.

Pudendal Nerve Innervates the external urethral and

anal sphincters and the pelvic and urogenital diaphragm muscles; it is part of the voluntary nervous system.

Radiation Therapy X-ray or other high-energy radiation treatment to destroy malignant, cancerous tissue.

Radical Prostatectomy Complete removal of the prostate gland, often used to treat prostate cancer.

Rectocele A bulging of the rectum into the posterior vaginal wall.

Rectum Final several inches of the intestines below the colon and above the anus.

Reflex Incontinence Loss of urine due to hyperactivity of the bladder muscle and/or involuntary urethral relaxation in the absence of the sensation associated with the desire to urinate. This occurs in neurogenic disorders.

Sphincter Circular muscle that tightens and relaxes to control the flow of urine from the urethra. There are internal and external urethral and anal sphincters.

Stress Incontinence Loss of small amounts of urine with increased intra-abdominal pressure during coughing, sneezing, laughing, jumping, running.

Testicles Two glands that produce sperm and sex hormones including testosterone in males (testes).

Testosterone Male sex hormone that is responsible for male sexual characteristics.

Trigone Base of bladder, near bladder neck that is most sensitive area of bladder.

Tumor Body mass caused by abnormal cell growth.

Ultrasound High-frequency sound waves used for medical diagnosis and treatment. An ultrasound scan (sonogram) is sound waves reflected off internal organs to produce computer-enhanced pictures of the bladder, prostate, and urethra.

Urethra Tube connecting the bladder to the outside through which urine is released.

Urethrocele Bulging of the urethra into the vaginal wall.

Urge Incontinence Sudden leaking of relatively large amounts of urine when the bladder muscle contracts, overcoming the contractions of the pelvic and urogenital diaphragm and sphincter muscles.

Urinalysis Tests on urine to diagnose diseases and infections.

Urinary Retention Quantities of urine backing up in the bladder which can cause bladder and kidney damage.

Urinary Tract Infection (UTI) Inflammation or infection in the bladder.

Urogenital Diaphragm Muscles that form the platform for the clitoris; the vagina and urethra pass through it.

Urologist Physician specializing in disorders of the urinary system.

Urology Specialty area of medicine dealing with the disorder of the urinary system.

Uterine Prolapse Descent of the uterus into the vaginal canal.

Uterus Muscular hollow organ that houses the fetus during pregnancy.

Vagina Elastic canal extending from the uterine cervix to the outside. Vaginal walls usually touch but can greatly expand, such as during childbirth.

X-rays Subatomic high energy particle of short wave length that penetrate body tissues to produce photographic images for diagnostic purposes.

ORDER FORM

Geriatric Incontinence: A Behavioral & Exercise Approach to Treatment	____ @ $29.95	= $_____
Beyond Kegels Book II: A Clinicians Guide	____ @ $85.95	= $_____
Beyond Kegels: Fabulous Four (Book I)	____ @ $14.95	= $_____
Physiological Quieting Tape	____ @ $10.00	= $_____
Physiological Quieting CD	____ @ $15.00	= $_____
Beyond Kegels Videotape	____ @ $49.00	= $_____
Personal Care Kit	____ @ $39.00	= $_____
Fibromyalgia: A Handbook for Self Care & Treatment	____ @ $14.95	= $_____

Please send check or money order to:

Phoenix Publishing
P.O. Box 8231
Missoula, MT 59807
1-800-549-8371

Subtotal $_____

Shipping/Handling
(7% of subtotal) $_____

TOTAL cost of order $_____

Name _____

Address _____

_____

City_____ State_____ Zip _____

Telephone (_____) _____